Mental Health Care for Nurses

Applying mental health skills
in the general hospital

Edited by

Anthony Harrison
Consultant Nurse in Liaison Psychiatry,
    Avon & Wiltshire Mental Health Partnership NHS Trust
Research Fellow, Faculty of Health & Social Care,
    University of the West of England

and

Chris Hart
Nurse Consultant in Liaison Psychiatry,
    South West London & St George's Mental Health NHS Trust
Principal Lecturer, Faculty of Health & Social Care Sciences,
    Kingston University & St George's Hospital Medical School

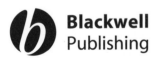
Blackwell
Publishing

© 2006 by Blackwell Publishing Ltd

Editorial offices:
Blackwell Publishing Ltd, 9600 Garsington Road, Oxford OX4 2DQ, UK
    Tel: +44 (0)1865 776868
Blackwell Publishing Inc., 350 Main Street, Malden, MA 02148-5020, USA
    Tel: +1 781 388 8250
Blackwell Publishing Asia Pty Ltd, 550 Swanston Street, Carlton, Victoria 3053, Australia
    Tel: +61 (0)3 8359 1011

First published 2006 by Blackwell Publishing Ltd

ISBN-10: 1405124555
ISBN-13: 9781405124553

Library of Congress Cataloging-in-Publication Data

Mental health care for nurses : applying mental health skills in the general hospital / edited by Anthony Harrison and Chris Hart.
    p. ; cm.
  Includes bibliographical references and index.
  ISBN-13: 978-1-4051-2455-3 (pbk. : alk. paper)
  ISBN-10: 1-4051-2455-5 (pbk. : alk. paper)
  1. Psychiatric nursing.   2. Psychiatric hospital care.   3. Nurse and patient.
  I. Harrison, Anthony, 1961–.   II. Hart, Christopher, RGN.
  [DNLM: 1. Mental Health Services.   2. Hospitals, General.   3. In-patients–psychology.   4. Nursing Care–methods.   5. Psychiatric Nursing–methods.
6. Residential Facilities.   WM 30 M5449 2006]
RC440.M349 2006
616.89′0231–dc22

                                                                    2005019403

A catalogue record for this title is available from the British Library

Set in 10/12.5pt Palatino
by Graphicraft Limited, Hong Kong
Printed and bound in India
by Replika Press, Pvt, Ltd, Kundli

For further information on Blackwell Publishing, visit our website:
www.blackwellnursing.com

Contents

Foreword

The world is gripped by an epidemic that affects one in four people. It is a mostly silent epidemic, unlike infections such as HIV or bird flu that scream from the news bulletins, but it is no less deadly for that – and it is growing. It is the epidemic of mental illness. Major depression, the leading global cause of disability, ranks fourth in the ten leading causes of the burden of disease and is set to reach second place by 2020, according to the World Health Organization. A million people kill themselves every year, 24 million have schizophrenia, and 70 million are dependent on alcohol.

Such figures are mind-numbing in scale, but the picture is also overwhelming when we look at the United Kingdom. Depression is the country's most common cause of long-term sick leave – accounting for more lost working days than back pain, that great scourge of the general nurse and midwife. Suicide is the leading cause of death in men under 35.

No one claims that preventing and treating such disorders is easy, yet there is mounting evidence of the power of medication, social support and talking therapies. Many of these interventions are relatively low cost, but are denied to countless people in need. This treatment gap highlights the scandal of stigma, discrimination and denial that pervades the epidemic. And nowhere is the gap more glaring, ironically enough, than in general hospitals, which you logically might expect to be at the forefront of closing it.

As this admirable book demonstrates, hospital patients with pre-existing mental illness or problems triggered by their physical condition are liable to be labelled 'difficult' and to receive poorer care. People with mental health problems are more likely to develop physical illnesses than the general population, and mental health problems are a temporary or longer-term concomitant of many physical diseases. Depression is twice as common in general hospital patients, for example, while 25% of older patients have dementia compared with 5% of their peers in the population as a whole. To deny them good mental health care is to deprive them of comfort, dignity and the possibility of alleviating physical as well as psychological symptoms.

Individual health needs have never fitted neatly into medically defined pigeonholes. What makes this issue so interesting is the way in which our physical and mental, emotional and spiritual dimensions are so intertwined, indeed inseparable – it is what makes us human. The closer we look, the more meaningless and artificial the boundaries seem. But whether the presenting problem appears to be mental or physical, good mental health care should be the core of all good practice. Whatever your profession or speciality, these skills should be an essential part of your tool kit.

It took us a long time to recognise the blindingly obvious fact that the quality of communication and relationship between patient, family and staff is crucial. Since the 1970s, British nursing discourse has rightly been concerned with the nurse–patient relationship. Observations on the emotional labour integral to all nursing work, and the therapeutic potential of the relationship, were considered rather way out when first floated but have now become accepted doctrine. Despite some progress, however, the necessary skills are still shamefully lacking in those who have no mental health training, and psychological care remains an undervalued aspect of the general nursing and midwifery role.

This book, therefore, presents a challenge to all nurses to overcome the barriers it so cogently describes – and not only to nurses, since it rightly draws attention to the political, organisational and cultural structures that maintain the barriers, and thus places equal responsibility on the shoulders of policy-makers, service planners, managers and educators. Even better, though, these pages contain a wealth of information, practical advice and examples of good practice that bring improvements within every nurse's grasp. The skills can be learned, but first the attitudes must shift, and this book will surely help us take a big step in that direction.

World Health Organization (2001). *The world health report 2001. Mental health: new understanding, new hope*. WHO, Geneva. www.who.int

Jane Salvage RGN, BA, MSc, HonLLD
International nursing consultant and board member, Global Initiative on Psychiatry

Editors

Anthony Harrison
Consultant Nurse in Liaison Psychiatry, Avon & Wiltshire Mental Health
Partnership NHS Trust, Bath
Research Fellow, Faculty of Health & Social Care, University of the West of
England, Bristol

Chris Hart
Nurse Consultant in Liaison Psychiatry, South West London & St George's
Mental Health NHS Trust
Principal Lecturer, Faculty of Health & Social Care Sciences, Kingston
University & St George's Hospital Medical School, London

Contributors

Gina Bird
Consultant Nurse in Liaison Psychiatry, Somerset Partnership Health and Social Care Trust, Yeovil

Alison Blofield
Nurse Consultant in Self-harm and Suicide Prevention, Shropshire County Primary Care Trust, Shrewsbury

Bob Gardner
Consultant Nurse in Liaison Psychiatry/Self-harm,
Derbyshire Mental Health Services, Derby

Lyn Williams
Nurse Consultant (Liaison Psychiatry)
Tees & North East Yorkshire NHS Trust, Middlesbrough

Dedication

AH – for my mother
CH – for Brenda

Acknowledgements

We would like to thank Beth Knight, Amy Brown and Katharine Taylor at Blackwell Publishing for their support and patience. We are also indebted to a number of other people: our families, colleagues and friends; Jane Hegan for her input in the planning stages, as well as her contributions to Chapter 1. Bill Bruce-Jones, Maggie Crowe, David Hillier and Rachael Redman at the Royal United Hospital Bath, for their help, advice, comments and feedback, all of which have been invaluable; Mo Wiles at the University of the West of England, Bristol; Rachael Aitchison, who never tired of endless requests for advice and comment; Liz Bessant, a very special nurse and friend; and Jenny Elliot for help with the admin and her cheerfulness. Thanks also to Paul, Rachel, David, Nicola, Jyoti, Jennifer, John, Niruji and Norman (who keeps coming back) in the liaison psychiatry services at St. George's Hospital.

Introduction

This book provides the essential foundations for truly patient-centred care. It aims to give nurses working in the general hospital the skills, confidence and enthusiasm to meet the mental health needs of their patient group. Although it necessarily addresses theoretical aspects of mental health care, and provides clear, concise guides to common mental health problems and mental illness, the emphasis is on the practical: what happens between the nurse and patient. It details how to undertake assessments, actual interventions that are effective in the types of everyday situation in which nurses find themselves, and how to develop structures and systems that can support this work.

Nonetheless, this is not simply a text aimed at helping nurses provide improved care for general hospital patients who have a pre-existing mental health problem. It is much more than that. Its focus is the mental health needs of the hospital patient group in its widest sense and the essential premise is that addressing those can have a transformative effect on patients, their care and the wider environment. We recognise the many demands on nurses' time and that some of the work detailed here may seem daunting. However, to genuinely deliver holistic care and develop the nurse–patient relationship to its full therapeutic potential, it is necessary for individual nurses to embrace the techniques detailed here and for clinical teams and senior managers to help develop and maintain the supportive structures and systems to facilitate this.

Terminology

We have written about the person's mental health rather than psychological state or emotional wellbeing, terms that will be more familiar to hospital nurses through the literature. This was a deliberate choice, as mental health encompasses the full range on the continuum of health to illness. This mirrors the book's content in looking at such things as emotional wellbeing, thought processes and the absence of actual mental illness. It also recognises that people with serious mental illness are more likely to suffer physical illness and need hospital care, where that care can be poor in comparison to the rest of the hospital population, affected by stigma and discrimination.

A conscious decision was taken to avoid talking about 'psychiatry' and 'psychiatric illness' although when referring to conditions such as schizophrenia or depression, we have used terms such as 'illness' and 'mental disorder'. These are, however, more the province of the psychiatrist and, as this book is intended for a nursing audience, it will focus on nursing concerns. Moreover, when discussing issues such as depressive symptoms or low mood, these have been placed in the context of the patient's life experience and mental health. We hope the distinction is clear.

Throughout the book we refer to 'patients'. This is because research has shown that this is the term patients prefer, even if they are healthy women attending antenatal classes (Byrne *et al.*, 2000; Rild *et al.*, 2000). We have used the feminine gender whenever we have identified nurses specifically. This reflects the fact that more than 80% of nurses are women, that nursing is still labelled as 'women's work' and gender issues underline the power relations in the contemporary NHS just as much as the nurse–doctor relationship did in the fledgling hospital services, mirroring the Victorian patriarchal society in which they developed. In this context, if patients are referred to by gender, in the masculine, it is simply to avoid confusion.

Structure of the book

There will always be things left out of a book with this scope and ambition. We took a conscious decision not to write about the mental health needs of children. It is too large a subject for a single chapter and deserves more attention. Readers may also find an area of concern not covered here but will, hopefully, feel sufficiently motivated to hunt it down elsewhere. We have categorised many conditions for the ease of reading but are mindful we have patients and need to respond to their holistic needs.

The book follows a straightforward structure. The first part provides context, themes and issues that arise in a range of situations, such as a consideration of legal and ethical matters, managing challenging situations and behaviours, and breaking bad news. The second part looks at specific conditions and a nursing approach to them.

Reflecting this approach, the first chapter is, essentially, in two parts. The first explores recent changes to the nursing role and context of the provision of holistic care. It then outlines some of the practical, organisational and educational difficulties in meeting the mental health needs of patients. The second provides an overview of the mental health problems that nurses are likely to encounter in their patient group, details the assessment process and outlines the skills and knowledge required to meet their broader mental health needs.

Issues such as influences upon health and ill health are explored in Chapter 2. This includes a discussion about how personal beliefs and interpretations are shaped, as well as how people react and adapt to illness and injury. It moves on to outline nursing priorities for providing psychological care, including dealing with emotions.

Many nurses worry about legal and ethical issues in relation to mental health care. Chapter 3 provides a framework for assessing decision-making, capacity and competence, consent and offers a brief overview of relevant areas of the Mental Health Act 1983. Caring for the person displaying challenging behaviours is the subject of Chapter 4. This looks at issues such as the causes of challenging behaviours, what it is about them that affects us as nurses – and why – before exploring strategies for addressing this problematic area of our work. Little is more challenging than having to break bad news to patients and relatives. The theory and practice of this under-developed area of nursing are covered in Chapter 5, focusing on a guide to best practice.

Even in hospitals where there is a well established mental health liaison team, nurses are often unclear as to its role, what it has to offer and how it operates. We provide an overview of a model for a liaison mental health service and how this can work effectively within the general hospital in Chapter 6.

Part 2 of the book focuses on specific mental health problems and disorders, detailing how nursing care can be provided. Chapter 7 looks at depression and anxiety, outlining theoretical perspectives, as well as how to recognise depression and various forms of anxiety disorders. Assessment and treatment strategies are followed by principles for planning the care of the patient.

Self-harm and suicide prevention are described in Chapter 8. This looks at the scale of the problem, causes, attitudes towards patients who self-harm or attempt suicide, the important area of risk assessment and caring for the person who has self-harmed. Chapter 9 explores perinatal and maternal mental health, from the policy context, through the impact of mental illness on new mothers, to common perinatal mental health problems.

Caring for the person with a mental illness admitted to the general hospital is the focus of Chapter 10. It provides definitions and terminology as well as a range of background knowledge to this important subject area before detailing the principles of caring for this patient group. A broad picture of the health problems associated with alcohol and illicit drug use is provided in Chapter 11, while Chapter 12 looks at the care needs of older people with a range of mental health problems, including dementia and delirium, as well as issues such as the impact of ageism.

Finally, Chapter 13 explores some of the constraining influences on holistic practice. These are broken down into organisational, educational and institutional factors and the way they influence contemporary nursing. However, the chapter also examines some of the interpersonal challenges nurses might encounter in attempting to meet the mental health needs of the patient before going on to highlight how structural support mechanisms can be developed that can assist nurses in this important aspect of their work.

The essence of nursing is in the relationship between the nurse and patient, embodied in the holistic care that embraces the mental health needs of the patient, recognises these as being as important as the physical, and brings them together to enhance the patient's experience. We hope this book will make a small contribution in helping nurses develop their knowledge and skills, experience and confidence in this vital area.

References

Byrne, D.L., Amussen, T. & Freeman, J. (2000) Descriptive terms for women attending ante natal classes: mother knows best? *British Journal of Obstetrics and Gynaecology*, 107: 1233–1236.

Rild, C.W., Hayes, D. & Ames, D.J. (2000) Patient or client? The opinion of people attending a psychiatric clinic. *Psychiatric Bulletin*, 24: 247–250.

Part 1
The Principles of Mental Health Care in the General Hospital

Chapter 1
The Provision of
Holistic Care

Chapter aims

> ### This chapter will:
>
> - introduce the context for contemporary nursing care
> - provide an overview of mental health problems commonly experienced in the general hospital
> - describe the process of mental health assessment in the general hospital
> - outline the mental health needs of the patient and how these can be met within the context of the nurse–patient relationship
> - explore how structural support mechanisms can assist nurses in these aspects of their work.

Introduction

This chapter is, essentially, in two parts. The first explores some of the theory relating to, and the context of, holistic care and the nurse–patient relationship. It outlines some of the practical, organisational and educational issues involved in enabling nurses to meet the mental health needs of their patients. The second part provides clinical guidelines on mental health problems commonly encountered in the general hospital, alongside an identification of the processes involved in undertaking a baseline mental health assessment. This is followed by a discussion of the practicalities of the nurse–patient relationship. Written about extensively, it is this relationship that lies at the absolute core of the work nurses do. It is a complex and challenging process to make contact with people on a deep emotional level and requires very specific skills. This chapter emphasises that it is not an 'add on' to the physical care provided: therapeutic communications are the means by which nurses facilitate that relationship. A necessary focus on how this is delivered and supported is required, not just on the part of the individual nurse, but ward teams and senior managers as well. While focusing on the issues outlined above, other parts of this book will return to these themes and some of the associated difficulties are explored in more detail in Chapters 4 and 13.

The focus of nursing and its relationship to holistic care

Holistic care is underpinned by two basic assumptions:

- The individual always responds as a unified whole.
- Individuals as a whole are different from, and more than the sum of, their parts (Pearson *et al.*, 1997).

The *Oxford Concise Medical Dictionary* (1996) defines the term *holistic* as 'an approach to patient care in which the physical, mental and social factors in the patient's condition are taken into account, rather than just the diagnosed disease'. Thus, despite the apparent expansion of the nursing role, holistic care has proved to be largely incompatible with the practicalities of contemporary nursing. Another irony lies in the way the academic and theoretical base of nursing and nursing models is interpreted and implemented. On the one hand, a theory is

'a set of concepts, definitions and propositions that project a systematic view of phenomena by designing specific interrelationships among concepts for purposes of describing, explaining and predicting' (Chinn & Jacobs, 1987).

On the other hand for Henderson (1969):

'The unique function of the nurse is to assist the individual, sick or well, in the performance of those activities contributing to health or its recovery (or a peaceful death) that the patient would perform unaided if the patient had the necessary strength, will or knowledge, and to do so in such a way as to help the patient gain independence as rapidly as possible.'

Both imply a holistic approach, with the nurse attempting to meet all of the patient's needs. Going beyond the act of physically tending to the care needs of someone who is 'ill' or 'injured' and meeting the needs of the whole individual thus requires nurses to adopt a bio-psychosocial perspective and have the skill and ability to develop a therapeutic relationship. While Table 1.1 outlines the different stages of the nurse–patient relationship, Peplau (1969) stated this was demonstrated by the nurse 'bringing all her capacities, talents and competencies to bear upon the life of another person'. It requires a closeness, 'not so much . . . to the person who is ill, but rather one of being "closer to the truth" of that person's current dilemma'.

Peplau's (1969) view was that the nurse has to 'put herself aside', or remain detached to achieve this, learning particular skills to demonstrate concern, interest and competence. Subsequent authors have emphasised the importance of partnership, mutuality and reciprocity as being the key elements of the

Table 1.1 Stages in the development of the nurse–patient relationship.

Pre-orientation phase	Gathering data and information from all available sources
Environmental phase	Creating as safe and confidential an environment as possible
Orientation phase	Establishing a rapport and using a variety of skills to develop a therapeutic relationship within the available time, specific to the task and to facilitate the function of assessment
Working phase	Identifying elements critical to the patient's physical and psychological health and safety, as well as therapeutic elements which aid personal control and coping. Undertake a mental state assessment at this stage
Formulation	Identifying risk, unmet needs, adopt a problem solving approach, managing risk and detailing a clear rationale for actions taken
Termination	Liaising with other health care professional and carers, referrals to specialist agencies

Modified from Fortnash and Holoday-Worret (2000); Roberts and Mackay (1999).

ideal therapeutic relationship (Savage, 1995). When studying nurses' relationships with patients and the work they were doing, Smith (1992) concluded that caring does not come naturally, and that nurses have to develop themselves emotionally to appear to care, irrespective of their personal feelings about themselves, the patient, and the conditions and circumstances in which they work. In doing so, they can be taught to manage their emotions more effectively. Vitally, Smith understood that if this 'essential ingredient of what nurses do is to be recognised and valued [it must be] supported organisationally and educationally'.

The actual skills employed within the therapeutic relationship are explored later in this chapter, but Smith's observations aside, it is obvious that the evolution of the nursing role must be supported by changes in education and training, not only for pre-registration students but also for qualified nurses. Concerns have long been voiced about both, for example, by nursing's former regulatory body the United Kingdom Central Council for Nursing, Midwifery and Health Visiting (1999) and the Department of Health (DoH) (1999a). Educationalists, meanwhile, have struggled to prevent nurse education being steered too strongly by the short-term needs of the service. Continuing professional development programmes are also affected by the broader context of health care provision and are thus not immune from financial constraints or organisational, structural and policy changes. This makes holistic care more difficult, due to factors beyond the control of the nurses expected to do it, with funding problems and staffing shortages maintaining the discredited system of task allocation (Baly, 1980).

Nursing models might have seemed another way in which holistic care could be embedded into practice. Ersser and Tutton (1991) acknowledged 'the explicit reference to the broad humanistic and holistic principles underlying nursing models'. A model has been portrayed as 'a descriptive picture of practice which adequately represents the real thing', which can lead to greater consistency in patient care by providing a framework for the direction, understanding and delivery of that care (Pearson *et al.*, 1997). There are numerous models, but many have problems in meeting the mental health needs of patients in an acute hospital setting. This is exemplified through a brief examination of Roper, Logan and Tierney's *Activities of Living Model for Nursing* (2000), which comprises five major concepts:

- Activities of living (of which 12 types were identified)
- Lifespan
- Dependence/independence continuum
- Factors that influence an individual's activities of living (including psychological)
- Individuality in living

Based upon an assessment of the 12 activities of daily living listed in the first concept, the nurse can utilise a focused approach to the planning, implementation and evaluation of the patient's care from admission through to discharge. Integral to the model is the notion that the nurse gets to know the patient and understand him as an individual. However, many nurses using it remain activity focused and often neglect the more complex and less easily accessed elements of the fourth major concept, when the individual's psychological needs are explicitly identified.

The context of care: mental health in the general hospital

The general hospital nurse will face large numbers of patients presenting with a wide variety of mental health conditions. Ramirez and House (1997) identified three main types of mental health-related clinical problem:

(1) Acute primary psychiatric disorder including:
  (a) self-harm
  (b) psychiatric crises and emergencies
(2) Psychiatric disorder in patients with any type of physical illness[1]
(3) Psychologically based physical symptoms, e.g. somatisation (Harrison, 2001).

---

[1] This should be taken to include co-existing mental illness, e.g. schizophrenia or mental health problems as a result of physical illness such as adjustment disorder and depression.

More than half a century ago, in *The Work of Nurses in Hospital Wards* (Goddard, 1953) it was noted that there was difficulty in meeting specific patient needs in isolation, and task allocation meant that little time was given to emotional care (White, 1985). The evidence suggests little has changed. Benjamin *et al.* (1994) estimate that between 20% and 40% of all people referred or admitted to the outpatients department of a general hospital will have psychological disorders or mental health problems in addition to the physical disorders that prompted their original referral or admission. It has also been estimated that between 20% and 30% of those attending emergency departments will have mental health problems co-existing with physical disorders and 5% will have presented due to mental health problems alone (Royal College of Physicians/Royal College of Psychiatrists, 1995; Storer, 2000). Yet the mental health needs of patients who are admitted into the general hospital often remain overlooked or ignored. For example, while 11% of all medical inpatients are depressed, only 50% of depression is actually recognised on medical wards (Feldman *et al.*, 1987).

This difficulty in recognising and responding to such high rates of psychological morbidity in general hospitals not only presents a challenge in itself, but it also reflects older dualistic concepts of philosophers such as Descartes, who conceived the idea of the separation of mind and body (Turp, 2001). This is exemplified in the artificial divide between physical and mental health services at educational, organisational and funding levels, with serious consequences for individual patients and families, as well as the service as a whole (Box 1.1; see Chapter 2).

Although numerous policies such as the *National Service Framework for Mental Health Services* (DoH, 1999b) or national guidelines for self-harm (National Institute for Clinical Excellence, 2004) fail to identify any structure or

---

Box 1.1 Potential consequences of psychological conditions being unrecognised.

- Decrease in the quality of life of the patient, and possibly their relatives/carers
- Physical recovery will often be affected
- Longer inpatient stay in hospital can lead to further physical investigations in a search for 'answers' which may not be necessary
- Cost implications for the National Health Service (NHS) as a result of lengthy inpatient stays and associated treatments
- A longer period off work and related financial problems as a result
- Social isolation
- Severity of mental health problems can be increased
- Higher risk of suicide

(Robinson *et al.*, 1986; Robinson, 1987; Egan-Morriss *et al.*, 1994; Mayou, 1995; Maguire & Haddad, 1996; Morriss, 1999; Mayou *et al.*, 2000)

Table 1.2 Summary of safety of clients/patients with mental health needs in acute mental health and general hospital settings (DoH, 2003).

Factor	Benchmark of best practice
Orientation to the health environment	All patients/clients are fully orientated to the environment, in order to help them feel safe
Assessment of risk of patients/clients with mental health needs harming self	Patients/clients have a comprehensive, ongoing assessment of risk to self with the full involvement of patient to reduce potential for harm
Assessment of risk of patients/clients with mental health needs harming others	Patients/clients have a comprehensive, ongoing assessment of risk to others with full involvement of patient to reduce potential for harming others
Balancing observation and privacy in a safe environment	Patients/clients are cared for in an environment that balances safe observation and privacy
Meeting patients'/clients' safety needs	Patients/clients are regularly and actively involved in identifying care that meets their safety needs
A positive culture to learn from complaints and adverse incidents	There is a no blame culture which allows a vigorous investigation of complaints and adverse incidents and near misses and ensures that lessons are learnt and acted upon

requirements for the provision of mental health care in the general hospital, *Essence of Care* (DoH, 2003) does provide a mental health benchmark, 'The safety of clients/patients with mental health needs in acute mental health and general hospital settings', and offers a framework for establishing and monitoring standards of mental health care. This benchmark enables practitioners, patients and carers to influence and participate in developing best practice that is linked to comparison and sharing. It is one of eight benchmarks that focus on fundamental aspects of care, developed after feedback from patient groups, identification of recurring themes from the ombudsman's complaints and analysis of common complaints from mental health service users (see Table 1.2).

The *Essence of Care* initiative is still being implemented across the UK, but strategic health authorities have been set targets for implementation that bring together senior hospital and mental health personnel. If a meaningful dialogue can be established, this offers the possibility of finally establishing an integrated approach to the care needs of the hospital population (Harrison & Devey, 2003; Harrison & Bessant, 2004).

Stigma and mental health in the general hospital

Apart from organisational difficulties, stigma also contributes to the problem of meeting the mental health needs of patients, marking an individual out as being different and evoking some form of sanction. While stigma related to illnesses such as cancer has declined, people with mental disorders remain some of the most stigmatised. Stigmatising beliefs often result in discrimination, and for people with mental illness, stigma is the largest single obstacle to improving their quality of life (Sartorius, 1998). The stigmatisation of mental illness among clinicians has been less studied than in the wider population, where it is acknowledged as being deep-seated (Royal College of Psychiatrists/Royal College of Physicians/British Medical Association, 2001). However, junior medical staff appear to have more negative and unrealistic attitudes towards mental illness than more senior colleagues (Mukherjee *et al.*, 2002) and a whole swathe of pejorative terms such as 'nutter' are still fairly common currency in organisations which are actively trying to stamp out other prejudices such as racism and sexism. More positively, as with any form of prejudice or ignorance, there is the implication that such attitudes may respond to education and training, which might explain the more positive attitudes of senior medical staff (Bolton, 2003).

The impact on nurses of meeting the mental health needs of the patient

It is not just negative attitudes and stigma that affect clinicians and their response to patients with psychological distress and mental health problems. Menzies' (1970) groundbreaking study of nurses and nursing in a London teaching hospital sought to explain how complex social systems were established as a means of defence against anxiety. Menzies discovered that the petty rules, traditions of behaviour and conduct, strongly hierarchical structures, and intricate dress codes were all designed to keep at bay the intense physical and, particularly, psychological discomfort that arose from caring for, and tending to, the sick and dying. The problem was, however, that such techniques were ineffective. Worse, because there were no mechanisms for recognising and addressing nurses' collective anxieties, these were displaced and added to the dysfunctional nature of the system in which they were working. Integral to this system had been task allocation, with the nurse–patient relationship fragmented. Decision-making was distant from the nurses delivering care, the workforce was de-personalised by such things as the use of the term 'nurse', responsibility was minimised by needless things like checking and counter-checking, avoidance of change and the denial of feelings. Menzies concluded that the unconscious anxieties persisted in a vague and debilitating fashion, contributing to the high number of nurses leaving the service.

However, as changes were made to the systems of nursing, little attention was paid to providing problem-solving mechanisms that would allow nurses to improve their working situation, and little in the way of clinical supervision that would allow them to articulate and work through the (often appropriate) anxieties and distress experienced as a consequence of more intense work with patients. In this context, nurses who were already operating within an 'increasingly de-humanised process [that is] the practice of medicine' (Cobbs, 1975), would inevitably find it even more difficult to care for overtly distressed and/or disturbed patients who would challenge them on almost every level. Although, as we have seen, there has been some reversion to tasks, little has been done to provide contemporary nurses with the necessary authority to match their levels of responsibility. Few have access to effective structures for problem-solving, such as shared governance, which engages them in addressing the practical issues they grapple with. Most receive little or no psychological support or clinical supervision, or even an acknowledgement that it is necessary, despite the intensity of their clinical work (Dartington, 1994). Meeting the mental health needs of their patients remains at least as difficult as it has in any of the preceding decades (Box 1.2).

Box 1.2 Summary of the factors that impact upon the nurse when addressing patients' psychological needs.

- Different elements of nursing care have now been segregated and are carried out by specialist staff, e.g. discharge co-ordinators
- The emphasis on more technology and competing organisational targets and needs create an environment where many hospital patients have shorter stays and the nurse has less time to develop a relationship
- Nursing models do not always relate to the psychological needs of the patient
- Many nurses perceive the busy physical demands and environments of the ward as not allowing them the time, opportunity or privacy to be able to deal with the patient's 'psychological needs', whereas addressing the activities of daily living fits well in that type of environment
- Nurses might be tempted to think it is 'not their job', or that they do not have the skills, to deal with patients' psychological problems (particularly if they have access to a mental health liaison service)
- A lack of understanding of the relationship between physical and psychological factors, and of a patient's psychological state and behaviour – particularly if this is challenging – can lead to resentment, with nurses feeling it is better for them to meet the 'real' physical needs of 'more deserving' patients
- The administrative burden has increased exponentially, with more documentation and more meetings for senior nursing staff to attend, removing them from the clinical area and which coincide with a far greater managerial role that limits their involvement in clinical work

Overview of mental health problems commonly encountered in the general hospital

This section cannot provide an exhaustive list of every mental health problem and psychiatric condition that will be found in patients with physical illnesses, but offers an overview of some of the most common conditions that nurses working with physically ill patients will encounter (Table 1.3).[2] Some are maladaptive responses to physical ill health, for example, adjustment disorders, while others may exist as co-morbid disorders, such as psychosis.

Most people become distressed in response to developing major health problems, particularly if this requires hospitalisation, where the environment is so different from their everyday experience, and often perceived as unpredictable and beyond their control (Royle & Walsh, 1992). Nurses and medical staff often – rightly – view this as being 'normal' and 'understandable' when physical illness is present and some of the conditions identified lie on a continuum between adaptive and maladaptive responses (see Chapter 2). Anxiety is a case in point, being a 'pervasive aspect of everyday life' (Stuart, 2001), and a basic survival response that is both necessary and normal (Rogers et al., 2004). Nonetheless, it is important that the nurse makes it a regular feature of her nursing care and relationship building with the patient that she finds time to talk with him about his individual emotional and psychological response to his illness. This allows for the patient reaction to be addressed over time and prevents a 'healthy' response developing into a more serious problem. In order for nurses to be able to do this they need have little more than a fundamental knowledge of different conditions and assessment techniques and of how to apply their nursing skills.[3]

It is important to remember that each individual's reaction is unique and influenced by a variety of factors, related to their illness or injury, personal characteristics and the health care environment (Moos, 1977). It is necessary, therefore, to assess each person as an individual and, wherever possible, discuss with them options for further care and treatment. Assessment will also help the nurse decide about further referral to specialist mental health staff within the hospital (see Chapter 6).

---

[2] Further information on most of these conditions, nursing care and treatment can be found in more depth in other chapters. Aspects of the nurse–patient relationship, assessment and care can also be found later in this chapter.

[3] The common psychiatric conditions described in this chapter are categorised, where appropriate, using the two main standardised criteria that are used for diagnosing psychiatric disorders – the International Classification of Diseases (ICD-10) (World Health Organization, 2003) and the Diagnostic and Statistical Manual (DSM-IV) (American Psychiatric Association, 1987).

Table 1.3 Summary of the mental health problems and mental illnesses commonly encountered in inpatients, people attending outpatient clinics and the emergency department.[4]

Condition	Presenting symptoms will include:	Treatment options include:
Adjustment disorder A maladaptive reaction in response to an identifiable event or situation that is stress-producing. Adjustment disorders occur in one quarter of general medical patients (Royal College of Psychiatrists/Royal College of Physicians, 1995)	Impaired social or occupational functioning that is more intense than the 'normal' expected response Reaction occurs within approximately three months of the stressor event Reduction of the reaction generally occurs when the identified stressor diminishes or is no longer present (i.e. resolves within six months of the cessation of the stressor or its effects) (Fortnash & Holoday-Worret, 2000)	Psychological interventions and social support, focusing on education and psychotherapeutic clarification of the individual's particular stressor or conflict (McDaniel et al., 2000)
Somatisation (medically unexplained symptoms) A condition where the person presents with a bodily symptom which has no organic cause, i.e. all medical investigations have ruled out an underlying physical cause. It may also be described as a medically unexplained symptom or symptoms (Harrison, 2001)	The most common symptoms are headache, back pain, abdominal pain, fatigue, chest pain, and dizziness (Kroenke & Mangelsdorff, 1989) Up to half the patients presenting with medically unexplained symptoms have underlying anxiety or depressive disorders which may pass unrecognised in a medical clinic (Katon et al., 1991) Distress, disability and panic attacks are common in patients with chronic somatisation	Cognitive behavioural approaches can be a successful treatment. If somatisation is quickly and correctly diagnosed, prognosis is good

---

[4] Self-harm, alcohol and drug misuse are dealt with in Chapters 8 and 11, respectively.

Anxiety

A feeling of apprehension, uncertainty and fear without apparent stimulus or an objective source of danger, associated with physiological changes It ranges from moderate to severe, with the latter often leading to progressive avoidance and withdrawal from the feared situations and stimuli A panic attack is a discrete period of intense fear or discomfort in which symptoms develop abruptly and peak within 10 minutes (Stuart, 2001)	Feelings of apprehension, discomfort, dread, fear, impending doom and panic. Physical symptoms include palpitations, diarrhoea, headache, nausea, frequency of micturition, increased respiration and muscle spasm Anxiety often co-exists with one or other psychiatric disorders and careful assessment and diagnosis is vital if the patient is to be treated appropriately	Psychological therapies, i.e. cognitive and behavioural therapies, anxiety management (involves relaxation techniques) and pharmacotherapy, i.e. benzodiazepine and antidepressant medications[5] A combination of medication and psychological therapies has also been found to be successful (National Institute for Clinical Excellence, 2004)

Hypochondriasis

A preoccupation with a persistent fear or belief of having a serious disease based on the individual's interpretation of physical sensations as signs of physical illness. This is rarely assuaged by positive results from physical examinations and tests	This will depend on the particular individual and may not be consistent with an actual illness or physiological responses	As with somatisation, cognitive behavioural therapy can be a successful treatment

Post-traumatic Stress Disorder (PTSD)

Classified as an anxiety disorder, occurring as a delayed psychological response – within six months – after an individual has been 'exposed to an extreme traumatic stressor involving actual or threatened death or serious injury, or a threat to the physical integrity of self or others' (Rogers et al., 2004). The individual will have experienced intense fear, pervasive distress and helplessness The vast majority of individuals exposed to a traumatic event will adapt, with only a small percentage developing PTSD. In the first month following the event it is very difficult to differentiate from a normal reaction which includes a grief reaction, e.g. loss of a limb following an accident	Repetitive, intrusive recollection or re-enactment of the event in memories, daytime imagery or dreams Conspicuous emotional detachment and numbing of feelings Avoidance of stimuli or activities that may arouse recollection of trauma is often present, but this symptom is not essential for a diagnosis to be made Hyper-arousal, manifesting as irritability, panic attacks and hyper-vigilance	Some models of psychotherapy such as cognitive therapy, family therapy, behavioural therapy and psychodynamic therapy Antidepressant medication NB: No positive effect has been shown for individual brief psychological intervention and some trials have even shown a worse outcome (Davidson, 1997; Wessely et al., 2000)

---

[5] Benzodiazepines such as diazepam and lorazepam are intended for short-term management of generalised anxiety disorder (2–4 weeks duration only) but not panic disorders. Certain antidepressants have also been successfully used in the treatment of anxiety.

Table 1.3 (*Cont'd*)

Condition	Presenting symptoms will include:	Treatment options include:
Depression Diagnosed when a patient's mood is consistently depressed or there is loss of interest and pleasure for at least two weeks and accompanied by four or more other symptoms from those listed in the next column. Physical illnesses such as cancer, respiratory and cardiovascular disease, diabetes, stroke and neurological conditions increase the risk of depression. Similarly, depression following a cerebral vascular accident, myocardial infarction or prolonged physical illness is associated with increased mortality (Robinson et al., 1986; Robinson, 1987; Egan-Morriss et al., 1994; Mayou, 1995; Maguire & Haddad, 1996; Morriss, 1999; Mayou et al., 2000) Symptoms of depression can be difficult to identify in physically ill patients as they are often the same as symptoms of the physical illness and associated treatments such as medication, chemotherapy, radiotherapy, etc. (e.g. changes in sleep and appetite). It is therefore important to focus upon the further assessment of the psychological symptoms	Feelings of worthlessness or guilt Impaired concentration Loss of energy/fatigue Suicidal thoughts Appetite/weight change Altered sleep pattern Tearfulness Depressive body posture Retardation Agitation Social withdrawal Inability to be 'cheered up'	Treatment can include medication (antidepressants), psychological interventions, social support and physical care if this is compromised (National Institute for Clinical Excellence, 2004)
Psychotic disorder A 'severe mental disorder in which the person's ability to recognise reality and his or her emotional responses, thinking processes, judgement and ability to communicate are so affected that his or her functioning is seriously impaired' (Warner, 1994)	Positive symptoms, including: Delusions, or false beliefs, firmly held, despite objective and contradictory evidence Hallucinations – false sensory perceptions, or perceptual phenomena arising without any external stimuli, e.g. hearing (most common), seeing, smelling, feeling or tasting things that other people do not	Psychosocial interventions Stress reduction Antipsychotic medication

Thought disorders, or interference with thinking
Anxiety
Negative symptoms, including:
Blunted emotions, social withdrawal, cognitive deficits and apathy

Eating disorders

Conditions in which there is excessive preoccupation and concern with control of body weight and shape, with grossly restricted food intake (Basu, 2004)

Most patients in a general hospital with conditions such as anorexia nervosa or bulimia nervosa will have been admitted for physical problems related to the eating disorder

An eating disorder may also be found in patients admitted with another condition or illness. It may also be a factor to consider in patients with medically unexplained symptoms, e.g. weight loss, vomiting, abdominal or menstrual complaints (Sharpe & Peveler, 1996)

Eating disorders are more prevalent in industrialised countries where food is plentiful and 'being thin' is considered attractive. There are 14.6 cases of anorexia per 100 000 per year in females and 1.8 cases per 100 000 per year in males. Only one in ten bulimia sufferers seeks help and is having treatment to overcome the condition. The onset of eating disorders is most common in adolescents and up to 90% of both anorexia and bulimia sufferers are female. The prognosis for eating disorders varies widely. Steinhausen (2002) found that 50% of patients with anorexia still never fully recover with overall mortality at 5%, while 20% of patients stay chronically ill

Anorexia nervosa
Failure to maintain minimum weight for age and height
Determined food avoidance
Extreme fear of gaining weight
Disturbed perceptions of self, i.e. sees self as fat even when very underweight
In females, amenorrhoea in post-menarcheal adolescents or delayed or arrested puberty (Basu, 2004)

Bulimia nervosa
Repetitive episodes of binge eating, i.e. uncontrollably eating a large quantity of food in a defined period of usually less than two hours
Intense craving for and/or preoccupation with food and overeating
Methods to prevent weight gain, i.e. self-induced vomiting, the misuse of laxatives and/or diuretics and excessive exercise
Intense preoccupation with body weight and shape

Specialist mental health teams will provide a wide range of treatments for people with eating disorders, including individual and group psychotherapy, cognitive behavioural therapy, and pharmacological treatments

The issue of re-feeding the patient is highly emotive and raises a number of ethical and legal issues. It is, however, the only time that the Mental Health Act 1983 can be used to physically treat someone but should only be used in life-threatening situations

In most cases, the patient will already be linked with mental health services. The clinical team should utilise their mental health colleagues' experience and knowledge of the patient in order to provide consistency with the overall management plan, particularly around eating and meal times, boundary setting and physical care

Table 1.3 (*Cont'd*)

Condition	Presenting symptoms will include:	Treatment options include:
Mental health problems are common in eating disorder sufferers. Depression and obsessive compulsive characteristics are often found in eating disorder patients, particularly in anorexia. Low self-esteem, impulsivity, conflicts with intimacy and dependency, and difficulty managing anger are common traits in bulimia patients There is a range of medical complications that can be experienced. These affect all body systems but, in addition to amenorrhoea, osteoporosis, hypometabolic symptoms such as cold intolerance, bradycardia, hypotension and constipation will be common in patients with anorexia nervosa. In bulimia nervosa, gastric, oesophageal and bowel abnormalities, hypokalaemia and potassium depletion are common, the latter causing muscle weakness, cardiac arrhythmias and hypotension (Cochrane, 2001)		Ongoing assessment can be provided by the mental health team and it may be beneficial to have a registered mental health nurse with the patient continuously if she or he is deemed to be high risk
Dementia (see also Chapter 12) A cluster of symptoms that provide a label for a range of specific behavioural, psychological, physical and social deficits. The incidence increases dramatically with age but tends to be rare in the under 55 age group (Longmore *et al.*, 2002). The commonest form of dementia is Alzheimer's disease, which accounts for 50–70% of all cases. The onset is insidious and irreversible. The disease progresses gradually but continuously and survival is approximately 8–11 years from the time of onset of symptoms Other primary causes of dementias include: Huntington's chorea (hereditary disease caused by a defect in a single gene)		Person-centred nursing is key to the care and treatment of patients with dementia (Morton, 1999). Pharmacological treatments with anticholinesterases are also now being used – see Chapter 12 for more detailed information

Pick's disease (rare form of dementia affecting the frontal and temporal lobes of the brain)
Creutzfeld–Jakob disease
There are many other causes of dementia of a secondary nature:
Brain tumours (primary and metastatic brain tumours)
Korsakoff's disease (alcohol dementia)
Trauma (head injury)
Drugs
Infection (e.g. HIV/AIDS)
Hydrocephalus

Delirium (see also Chapter 12)

Characterised by a transient and fluctuating mental state. It is a reversible medical condition of organic cause although it has neuro-psychiatric aspects which may require specialist psychiatric advice in terms of management of associated behaviours

Delirium is more common after 60 years of age, and it is detected in at least 10% of those admitted to hospital with acute illness (Lipowski, 1987)

Causes of delirium include:
Infection
Drugs (sedatives, anticonvulsants, opiates, etc.)
Stroke
Myocardial Infarction
Hypoxia
Hypoglycaemia
Liver failure
Thiamine or B_{12} deficiency
Alcohol withdrawal
Trauma
Epilepsy
Pain
Encephalitis/meningitis

Impaired consciousness, which can occur over hours or days
Disorientation to time, place and person
Erratic behaviour
Thinking can be slow and muddled
Paranoia is also common
Perception is usually disturbed, with illusions and visual or tactile hallucinations common
Mood is often labile, ranging through anxiety, depression and agitation
Memory is impaired. After the episode of delirium is over, the person often cannot remember it

The cause of the delirium should be treated (e.g. any infection) and, while nurses can address the affect associated with it (e.g. anxiety, fear, etc.), in extreme cases, where the patient is at risk, psychotropic medication can be used – see Chapter 12 for more detailed information

Mental health assessment

Assessment has four overall objectives (Barker, 1997):

■ Measurement – gaining information on the scale or size of a problem.
■ Clarification – understanding the context or conditions of the problem.
■ Explanation – exploring the possible cause, purpose or function of the problem.
■ Variation – exploring how the problem varies over time, its seriousness and how it affects the individual.

Mental health screening and assessment tools are available to assist in assessment, and commonly used instruments include the Hospital Anxiety and Depression Rating Scale (Zigmond & Snaith, 1983), devised to determine the patient's levels of anxiety and depression in non-psychiatric hospital clinics, while the General Health Questionnaire (Goldberg, 1972) can be used to identify individuals suffering from non-psychotic mental health problems in general populations.

Neither aims to provide a diagnosis but rather to identify those in need of further assessment. Once the information has been gathered, and a problem identified, then it has to be used and appropriate action taken, which may include referral on to mental health services for a full mental health assessment. However, in most cases, it is appropriate that the ward team undertake a fuller assessment of its own before considering referral. First, any mental health problems identified might be within the competence and experience of the team to address. Second, this will allow a clearer discussion with the mental health liaison team if a referral is to be made (see Chapter 6).

There is obviously a difference between an assessment that a mental health nurse would undertake and that which might be expected of a nurse without any formal mental health training. The purpose of a more complete assessment is to comprehend the way in which a person functions as a result of their condition, the way in which their current problems affect them and ways in which they usually solve the problems, and adapt and employ their psychological strengths. Exploring the relationships between the person's thoughts, feelings and behaviour is a diagnostic process that nurses can, and do, perform well (Ryrie & Norman, 2004). It will also enable the nurse to help the patient make sense of his relationship with the external world and, in this case, the clinical team on the ward, as well as help the nurse determine whether or not the patient has the capacity to make informed decisions. Key components that constitute a baseline mental state assessment are outlined in Table 1.4.

A biographical history should, routinely, have been gathered at the time of admission, either by the doctor or by a nurse. This provides an opportunity to give an account of his personal and family history and how the current events fit within this. However, this is often not done. Not only is it unacceptable in the twenty-first century that people are under the care of clinical teams whose members know very little about them as individuals rather than a set

Table 1.4 Factors to consider when undertaking an assessment of the patient's mental health in a general hospital setting.

Factors to consider before assessment	Has a physical cause for the problem(s) been ruled out? Has drug and/or alcohol intoxication, or withdrawal, been ruled out as a cause? Is the person physically well enough (e.g. not sedated, intoxicated, vomiting or in pain) to interview? Does the person have a known mental health history? If so, is his mental health team involved in his care while he is in hospital?
History of presenting complaint, or what has prompted the assessment at this time	What recent event(s) precipitated or triggered this presentation or made you think assessment was necessary now? Does the person pose an immediate (i.e. within the next few minutes or hours) risk with specific plans to self-harm or aggression/violence towards you or others? Is there any suggestion, or does it appear likely, that the person may try to abscond?
Appearance and behaviour	Is the person obviously distressed, markedly anxious or highly aroused? Is the person quiet and withdrawn? Is the person behaving inappropriately to the situation? Is the person attentive and engaged with the assessment process? How does the patient look? This is best done as a photo shot description, e.g. clean shaven, dishevelled, make up worn, colour of hair, smiling How does the patient respond to and interact with the assessor? Does he make eye contact?
Biographical history	This comprises a personal, family and social history of the person, allowing him to tell his 'story' and placing his illness and current psychological/mental health problems in context It can include details about his financial and social situation, employment, social and sexual relationships[6]
Past psychiatric history	Does he have a history of violence? Has the person got a history of self-harm? Does the person have a history of mental health problems or psychiatric illness?
Speech	Is the speech slow, rapid, loud or very soft, disjointed, vague and lacking any meaningful content? Is the individual skipping from one subject to another? Is the speech 'pressured' (a rush of words that is difficult to stop)?

---

[6] A relevant issue many nurses find difficult to ask about is whether or not the individual has ever felt they have been abused, physically, emotionally or sexually. It may be that you do not feel confident to ask this but it is a valid and important line of enquiry.

Table 1.4 (*Cont'd*)

Thought content	What are the themes emerging from the patient's thoughts throughout the interview?
	Does the patient experience negative, obsessive or unwanted, intrusive thoughts?
	Delusional thoughts may also be present or other psychotic ideas (see Chapter 10)
	What does he think about his illness, treatment and prognosis?
Mood	How does the patient describe his mood?
	How do you see the patient's mood? The descriptions can be different, i.e. the patient may say that his mood is 'fine' or 'okay' (subjective) but the assessor may observe in the interview that the patient's mood is 'low' 'depressed' 'high' etc. (objective)
Perceptions	Does the person appear to be experiencing any delusions or hallucinations (see Chapter 10)?
	Does the person have any unusual beliefs about his illness that are not congruent with the information given or his situation?
	Does the person feel controlled or influenced by external forces?
Cognition	Does the person have the capacity to consent, i.e. can the patient understand and retain information, and then make balanced judgements based on an evaluation of his options?
	What is the patient's level of concentration?
Risk	Is the person at risk of:
	Suicide?
	Self-harm?
	Aggression and/or violence to others?
	Are there particular risks associated with the person's mental state and physical illness, e.g. hopelessness prompting non-adherence with treatment?
	Is the person at risk of self neglect?
	How immediate is the risk?
	What would be the likely impact of any actions if the person were to act upon his ideas?
Formulation	What is your understanding of the issues the patient has described?
	What is the level of risk?
	Is immediate action required?
	Is a referral to the liaison psychiatry team necessary?
	How urgent is the referral?

of symptoms and illness, but it is also very poor practice. There is now a large body of evidence that shows the patient's life experience is profoundly important in shaping such things as his health beliefs, attitudes to hospitalisation, social support and psychological strengths.

If there is a recognition that specialist assessment is going to be sought from the mental health liaison team, it may be better to undertake a truncated assessment, as the mental health nurse will need to go through a more detailed examination of the patient's mental state and related factors. However, as described in Chapter 6, basic information needs to be gathered before making a referral, including:

- the history of the presenting complaint and why the referral is being made at this time
- a summary of the patient's mental state
- any concerns about risk
- the urgency of the referral.

The nurse–patient relationship

As noted earlier in this chapter, both despite of and because of, the difficulties posed by a variety of organisational, educational and practice issues, there is a greater scope for nurses to utilise simple communications and interpersonal skills with patients experiencing mental health difficulties. The subject of the nurse–patient relationship has been well rehearsed in the literature. It is not the intention here to detail that but to provide the reader with an overview of its fundamental features in meeting the mental health needs of patients. We have looked at how a holistic approach to care involves integrating all aspects of the person's physical care needs with his psychological needs, which concerns his feelings, thoughts, beliefs and attitudes. It is then that the nurse is helping the patient to deal with his physical illness from a psychological and emotional viewpoint. Arnold and Underman-Boggs (1999) suggest that a therapeutic relationship requires a combination of full presence and emotional objectivity and describe it as:

> '*A conscious commitment on the part of the professional nurse to understand how an individual client and his/her family perceive, feel and respond to their world.*'

Rogers defined it as a 'helping relationship', characterised as one 'in which at least one of the parties has the intent of promoting the growth, development, maturity, improved functioning and improved coping with life of the other' (Sundeen *et al.*, 1998).

Benner and Wrubel (1989) claim that the presence of the nurse, both physically and psychologically, is significant for sustaining and deepening the relationship. The uniqueness of this, and the nature of the work it enables, is what then gives nursing its intimacy in comparison with the patient's relationships with other health professionals. Nurses are the only health workers actually providing care to – and with – patients around the clock. This is undoubtedly one of the reasons patients can 'connect' to the nurse as the one person in the health care team who can understand them from a 'holistic' perspective and thus communicate more empathically.

Such commitment by the nurse needs, however, to be visibly demonstrated and calls for the use of a range of interpersonal and communication skills, including Arnold and Underman-Boggs' notion of 'full presence' and 'emotional objectivity' (1999), self-awareness, emotional intelligence, reflection, critical thinking, and empathy. Again, it is not easy work and requires emotional labour (Smith, 1992) but, probably more than anything, gives nursing both its credibility and its authority.

Effective use of interpersonal skills and therapeutic communication

Hyland and Donaldson (1989) stated that the tool of psychological care is communication, as it is a fundamental requirement to understand what patients think and feel, and to develop a therapeutic relationship. McCabe (2004) argues that patient-centred communication is a basic component of nursing and facilitates the development of a positive nurse–patient relationship.

Although national guidance has effectively 'written out' nurses and nursing in the treatment and care of patients with anxiety and depression, or those who have self-harmed (National Institute of Clinical Excellence, 2004), this is more about the continued medical dominance of the policy agenda and a reliance on formal treatments, such as cognitive behavioural therapy, that few patients will access, particularly in the general hospital. Nonetheless, the use of therapeutic communications in nursing, empathy particularly, is what enables therapeutic change (Ryrie & Norman, 2004) and should not be underestimated.

Box 1.3 outlines the overall benefits of good communication, while Table 1.5 summarises particular skills that nurses can employ, although it needs to

---

Box 1.3 Overall benefits from positive and effective communications.

- Poor communication and unhelpful attitudes rate second highest in complaints against NHS trusts in DoH statistics (www.statistics.gov.uk)
- Effective communication with patients is related to positive outcomes. Explaining and understanding patient concerns even when they cannot be resolved results in a significant reduction in anxiety (Simpson *et al.*, 1991)
- Breaking difficult news to patients effectively ensures better adjustment and decreases the risk of the patient developing a mental health-related problem such as adjustment disorder or a mood disorder. It facilitates the use of coping strategies appropriately and decreases feelings of helplessness (Fallowfield *et al.*, 1990)
- Recognition of early signs of aggression or impending violence can help defuse angry or aggressive exchanges
- Failure of communication between staff members can put patients at risk and decrease the quality of working life for all disciplines involved

Table 1.5 Therapeutic communications.

Intervention	Explanation/example
Preparation (this is more for formal meetings)	
Use a quiet, private environment	Promotes confidentiality and minimises interruptions
Agree the agenda if necessary	Keeps the communication focused
Let the patient know how long you have for the interview	Allows both the nurse and patient to gauge the communications according to the time available. It can avoid the patient beginning to talk about very distressing issues just as the nurse has to go and do something else
Non-verbal	
Active listening	Repeating key words, affirming what has been said, making eye contact, helping the person elaborate on what they wish to say
Look for non-verbal cues	The patient may say everything is 'fine' but look depressed or tearful
Use – and tolerate – short silences	Allows both the nurse and patient to reflect on what has been said and its implications
Body language and posture	Physical congruence with what you are saying, making eye contact, and having a relaxed, open posture convey your interest in the person
Empathising with or recognition of *what* the other is feeling rather than *how* he or she is feeling	Conveyed by actively, or reflectively, listening and responding in a way that indicates an understanding of the patient's emotion and perspective, whether stated or not
Genuineness	Acting congruently to the situation, not over-emphasising the caring role. It is supported by being open and spontaneous, and not defensive
Verbal	
Use simple language with as little jargon as possible	Makes the communication process as straightforward as possible
Use open questions to encourage elaboration; also allows the patient to direct the interaction	'How do you feel about what's happened?'
Clarification	'I'm not sure what you mean. Could you tell me a bit more?'
Re-stating	'So you're saying that you find that difficult?'

Table 1.5 (*Cont'd*)

Intervention	Explanation/example
Engaging with the patient's agenda, or aligning	Finding out what the patient wants and why, e.g. how he wants to be cared for or treated
Set clear boundaries	Clarifying for the patient what are acceptable behaviours (as opposed to acceptable emotional responses)
Know how to close down the interview if you feel out of your depth or are not sure how to respond	'I can see this is distressing for you and I think it best that we pause at this time. It's not that I'm ignoring you, but my colleague, who is more skilled in this area, will talk some more with you about it.'
Summarising	Towards the end of the discussion, go over the key points again, and check whether or not the person wants further information, or to discuss anything in more detail
Confrontation	'Getting angry and shouting at the nurses doesn't help us understand how to help you. Can you say what you are actually concerned about?'
Problem solving	'I know this is very distressing for you but I wonder what might help or has helped you in similar situations?'

After the interview or discussion

Use diagrams	These can illustrate difficult technical concepts or anatomical information if the patient has difficulty understanding
Visual aids	These can be considered for people with a learning disability
The use of interpreters	Vital for anyone for whom English is their second language or who has a hearing disability when important communications are planned
Provide other sources of information, e.g. the internet, self-help organisations and leaflets	This might be a written record of the key points of the discussion, or even a tape. Leaflets from self-help or voluntary groups might be made available, as well as website addresses and anything else that might help the patient
Document, in detail, what has been discussed	Can be used as part of the feedback (also important to be done verbally) to the rest of the multi-disciplinary team

(Maynard, 1989; Buckman, 1992; Barker, 1997; Sundeen *et al.*, 1998; Russell, 2002; Ryrie & Norman, 2004) be remembered that the use of therapeutic communication techniques does not automatically guarantee therapeutic communication and, because of the many factors involved in human relationships, it is not possible to state that any particular skill, method or pattern of application guarantees success (Sundeen *et al.*, 1998). There are times when, for various reasons, a person cannot assimilate what is being said. This will often be displayed by the person not acknowledging or remembering the information given. Most important in such circumstances is for the nurse not to be deterred, but to look at how better communication can be facilitated, especially if what is required is to give the patient some space and time to reflect on what has been communicated.

These skills can obviously be utilised in more formal meetings with patients, for example, during an assessment or when preparing to impart or share bad news. However, most of them are highly applicable in any communication with the patient, even – indeed, especially – while the nurse is providing physical care. Other key characteristics the nurse can cultivate and exploit in communicating with patients, carers and relatives include altruism, courtesy, kindness, honesty and respect for others. Unconditional acceptance is communicated through accepting patients as people with needs entitled to care and respect (Russell, 2002). It is not to suggest that nurses do not make judgements or feel alienated from the behaviour or attitudes of some patients, but the act of caring comes, in part, from not revealing them.

Reflection and self-awareness can help the nurse consider her actions, their impact, or why care is being provided in the way it is, even questioning its necessity. Unnecessary care, like unnecessary tasks or 'being busy', takes valuable time away from qualitative interventions, such as those of therapeutic communication. Reflection and self-awareness also help the nurse understand why a particular intervention was selected and can help nurses avoid presumptive and ritualised practice (Jarvis, 1992). Equally, reflection can help guard against the widely advocated but ill-informed practice of giving 'reassurance', which conflicts with forms of care such as empathising and is often more about the nurse trying to assuage her own distress and uncomfortable feelings.

In reality, no one could demonstrate the above skills to patients at all times. As has been emphasised, it will always present a challenge to nurses, who will often have conflicting demands placed upon them, not only at work but also in their personal lives. Tiredness and stress affect the nurse's ability to communicate therapeutically and care effectively. Once more, self-awareness can enable the nurse to recognise this and take appropriate steps to adapt to it, possibly resolving the cause of the stress, possibly seeking the support of colleagues in not taking a lead in particularly difficult interactions or with patients she is finding challenging at that time. This necessarily requires good teamwork and a milieu where nurses can openly express their own vulnerability and concerns. It should be recognised that no nurse can work effectively outside such an environment (see Chapter 4).

Communication and recording of patient-related information

An essential part of communication concerns documentation. It is particularly important to avoid vague or potentially misleading terminology, labelling or jargon, all of which can create significant communication problems with the patient (see Chapter 4). Well written care plans, developed in negotiation with the patient wherever possible, will reflect the course of the patient's contact with nursing staff (Sundeen *et al.*, 1998), as well as the quality of that contact. Hackneyed phrases such as 'offer reassurance' or 'develop a therapeutic relationship' should be avoided. Specific interventions about communications and/or the patient's mental health needs or problems should be used, with interventions and objectives designed to address the problem or need identified.

It can take longer to document an interaction that explores an individual's mental health needs, but the key task is to convey what was communicated, from *both* sides, and should separate out a factual account of what occurred and the clinician's impression (although the latter may be important in itself). Documentation should include detailed information regarding the patient's presentation, identified mental health needs, results from the use of any screening or assessment tools, and a clear management plan. This should include a risk management plan describing who is responsible for each action (see Chapter 8).

Support mechanisms for nursing staff and other clinicians

A variety of mechanisms at different levels of the hospital organisation are required to enable nurses to perform the work outlined in this and other chapters. Organisational, educational and policy issues have already been touched upon. At ward level, a range of initiatives can be helpful. Ongoing training and education for the ward team on issues relevant to mental health and risk assessment can be provided, and many mental health liaison teams undertake this as a core element of their work (see Chapter 6).

Clinical supervision is a staff development process that aims to safeguard standards of care, facilitate personal and professional development and promote excellence in health care (Bishop, 1998). Research shows it has a beneficial impact on both patient care and staff health (Butterworth *et al.*, 1997), facilitates reflective practice and professional learning, and should be kept separate from managerial supervision – although it is important this is provided as well (Bond & Holland, 1998; Johns & Freshwater, 1998). Clinical supervision can be provided on a one-to-one basis or in groups, formally or informally. Whole-team training and supervision promote better quality decision-making, treatment and democratisation of work practices.

Another structural mechanism key to effective team working is shared governance. This is achieved through 'councils' made up of managers and clinicians from all backgrounds, all with equal authority, taking a solution focused approach to *all* aspects of the team's working, identifying its agenda from the staff affected by particular issues and where information is shared openly. This allows the team to address stressors that may be patient related or, more likely, to do with organisational issues, either within the team or wider hospital. Even if the whole team is not happy with the resolution of the issue, exerting influence and involvement in the process is still beneficial (DoH, 2001b).

Involving nurses in decisions around the admission of patients, discharge planning, treatment and care, rather than viewing this as the province of the medical team, also promotes the provision of holistic care in the most essential way. This can be achieved by regular clinical reviews involving clinicians from all disciplines rather than the traditional ward round.

Conclusions

This chapter has covered a lot of ground in outlining the elements of holistic care and the nursing approaches that can enable this. It is complex, difficult and often hampered by a range of external influences. It demands a lot of the individual nurse, the nursing team and others involved with the patient's care, in particular the multi-professional team, managers and educationalists. Paradoxically, it also makes demands of the patient. It requires managers and medical staff to relinquish some of their power and influence while nurses have to be prepared to develop their knowledge and skills, as well as expand the range of their nursing role. This is not achieved through picking up specific tasks that consume their time at the expense of core elements of their nursing role. As shall be seen throughout the remainder of this book, however, it is essential if the nurse is to be able to pro-actively meet the mental health needs of the patient.

References

American Psychiatric Association (1987) *Diagnostic and Statistical Manual of Mental Disorders*, 3rd edn. Washington: APA.

Arnold, E. & Underman-Boggs, K. (1999) *Interpersonal Relationships: professional communication skills for nurses*. Pennsylvania: W.B. Saunders.

Baly, M.E. (1980) *Nursing and Social Change*. London: Heinemann.

Barker, P. (1997) *Assessment in Psychiatric and Mental Health Nursing: in search of the whole person*. Cheltenham: Nelson Thornes Ltd.

Basu, R. (2004) Mental health problems in childhood and adolescence. In: I. Norman & I. Ryrie (eds) *The Art and Science of Mental Health Nursing*. Maidenhead: Open University Press.

Benjamin, S., House, A. & Jenkins, P. (1994) *Liaison Psychiatry: defining needs and planning services*. London: Gaskell.

Benner, P. & Wrubel, J. (1989) *The Primacy of Caring*. London: Addison-Wesley.

Bishop, V. (1998) Clinical supervision: what's going on? Results of a questionnaire. *Nursing Times Research*, 3 (2): 141–152.

Bolton, J. (2003) How can we reduce the stigma of mental illness? *BMJ Career Focus*, 326: 57.

Bond, M. & Holland, S. (1998) *Clinical Supervision for Nurses*. Buckingham: Open University Press.

Buckman, R. (1992) *How To Break Bad News: a guide for health-care professionals*. London: Papermac.

Butterworth, T., Carson, J. & White, J. (1997) *It's Good to Talk. An evaluation of clinical supervision and mentorship in England and Scotland*. Manchester: Manchester University Press.

Chinn, P.L. & Jacobs, M.K. (1987) *Theory and Nursing: a systematic approach*. St Louis: Mosby.

Cobbs, P.M. (1975) The victim's perspective. In: J. Howard & A. Strauss (eds) *Humanising Health Care*. Berkeley: University of California Press.

Cochrane, C.E. (2001) Eating regulation responses and eating disorders. In: G.W. Stuart & M.T. Laraia (eds) *Principles and Practice of Psychiatric Nursing*. St Louis: Mosby.

Davidson, J.R. (1997) Biological therapies for PTSD: an overview. *Journal of Clinical Psychology* 58 (suppl 9): 29–32.

Davidson, J.R., Kudler, H.S. & Saunders, W.B. (1993) Predicting response to amitriptyline in PTSD. *American Journal of Psychiatry*, 150: 1024–1029.

Dartington, A. (1994) Where angels fear to tread: idealism, despondency and inhibition in thought in hospital nursing. In: A. Obholzer & V. Zagier-Roberts (eds) *The Unconscious at Work: individual and organisational stress in the human services*. London: Routledge.

Department of Health (1999a) *Making a Difference*. London: DoH.

Department of Health (1999b) *National Service Framework for Mental Health Services*. London: DoH.

Department of Health (2000) *The NHS Plan*. London: DoH.

Department of Health (2001a) *Improving Working Lives*. London: DoH.

Department of Health (2001b) *Shifting the Balance of Power*. London: DoH.

Department of Health (2003) *Essence of Care: patient-focused benchmarks for clinical governance*. London: DoH.

Dexter, G. & Wash, M. (1990) *Psychiatric Nursing Skills: a patient-centred approach*, London: Chapman & Hall.

Egan-Morriss, E., Morriss, R. & House, A. (1994) The role of the nurse in consultation-liaison psychiatry. In: S. Benjamin, A. House & P. Jenkins (eds) *Liaison Psychiatry: defining needs and planning services*. London: Gaskell.

Ersser, S. & Tutton, E. (1991) *Primary Nursing in Perspective*. Middlesex: Scutari Press.

Fallowfield, L., Hall, A. & Maguire, P. (1990) Psychological outcomes of different treatment policies in women with early breast cancer outside a clinical trial. *British Medical Journal*, 301: 575–580.

Feldman, E., Mayou, R. & Hawton, K. (1987) Psychiatric disorder in medical inpatients. *Quarterly Journal of Medicine*, 63: 405–412.

Fortnash, K.M. & Holoday-Worret, P.A. (2000) *Psychiatric Nursing Care Plans*. Missouri: Mosby.

Goddard, H.A. (1953) *The Work of Nurses in Hospital Wards (The Goddard Report).* London: Nuffield Provincial Hospitals Trust.

Goldberg, D.P. (1972) *The Detection of Psychiatric Illness by Questionnaire: a technique for the identification and assessment of non-psychotic psychiatric illness.* London: Oxford University Press.

Harrison, A. (2001) Somatisation. *Mental Health Practice,* 4 (6): 31–38.

Harrison, A. & Devey, H. (2003) Benchmarking mental health care in a general hospital. *Nursing Times,* 99 (24): 34–36.

Harrison, A. & Bessant, L. (2004) Making time to benchmark practice. *Professional Nurse,* 19 (10): 6–7.

Henderson, V. (1969) *Basic Principles of Nursing Care.* Geneva: International Council of Nurses.

Hyland, M.E. & Donaldson, M.L. (1989) *Psychological Care in Nursing Practice.* Middlesex: Scutari Press.

Jarvis, P. (1992) Reflective practice in nursing. *Nurse Education Today,* 12: 178–181.

Johns, C. & Freshwater, D. (1998) *Transforming Nursing Through Reflective Practice.* Oxford: Blackwell Science.

Katon, W.J., Buchwald, D.S. & Simon, G.E. (1991) Psychiatric illness in patients with chronic fatigue and those with rheumatoid arthritis. *Journal of General Internal Medicine,* 6: 277–285.

Kroenke, K. & Mangelsdorff, A.D. (1989) Common symptoms in ambulatory care: incidence, evaluation, therapy and outcome. *American Journal of Medicine,* 86: 262–266.

Lipowski, J. (1987) Delirium, acute confusional states. *Journal of the American Medical Association,* 258: 1789–1792.

Longmore, M., Wilkinson, I. & Török, E. (2002) *Oxford Handbook of Clinical Medicine,* 4th edn. Oxford: Oxford University Press.

Maguire, P. & Haddad, P. (1996) Psychological reactions to physical illness. In: E. Guthrie & F. Creed (eds) *Seminars in Liaison Psychiatry,* pp. 157–191. London: Gaskell.

Maynard, D. (1989) Notes on the delivery and reception of diagnostic news regarding mental disabilities. In: D.T. Helm, T. Anderson & J.A. Meehan (eds) *Directions in the Study of Social Disorder.* New York: Irvington.

Mayou, R. (1995) Improving psychological care of cancer patients. In: A. House, R. Mayou, C. Mallinson *et al.* (eds) *Psychiatric Aspects of Physical Disease.* London: Royal College of Physicians Publication Unit.

Mayou, R.A., Gill, R. & Thompson, D.R. (2000) Depression and anxiety as predictors of outcome after myocardial infarction. *Psychosomatic Medicine,* 62: 212–219.

McCabe, C. (2004) Nurse–patient communication: an exploration of patients' experiences. *Journal of Clinical Nursing,* 13 (1): 41–49.

McDaniel, J.S., Brown, F.W. & Cole, S.A. (2000) Assessment of depression and grief reactions in the medically ill. In: A. Stoudemire, B.J. Fogul & D.B. Greenberg (eds) *Psychiatric Care of the Medical Patient,* 2nd edn. Oxford: Oxford University Press.

Menzies, I.E.P. (1970) *The Functioning of Social Systems as a Defence Against Anxiety.* London: Tavistock.

Moos, R.H. (1977) *Coping with Physical Illness.* New York: Plenum.

Morriss, R.K. (1999) Physical illness and depressive disorders. *Opinion in General and Elderly Medicine* 8–12.

Morton, I. (1999) *Person-centred Approaches to Dementia Care*. Oxon: Winslow.

Mukherjee, R., Fialho, A. & Wijetunge, K. (2002) The stigmatisation of psychiatric illness: the attitudes of medical students and doctors in a London teaching hospital. *Psychiatric Bulletin*, 26: 178–181.

National Institute for Clinical Excellence (2004) *Self-harm: the short term physical and psychological management of self harm in primary and secondary care*. London: NICE.

Oxford Concise Medical Dictionary (1996) 4th edn. Oxford: Oxford University Press.

Pearson, A., Vaughan, B. & Fitzgerald, M. (1997) *Nursing Models in Practice*. Oxford: Butterworth Heinemann.

Peplau, H.E. (1969) Professional closeness. *Nursing Forum*, 8 (4): 342–360.

Ramirez, A. & House, A. (1997) Common mental health problems in hospital. *British Journal of Psychiatry*, 314: 1679–1682.

Roberts, D. & Mackay, G. (1999) A nursing model of overdose assessment. *Nursing Times* 95: 3.

Robinson, L. (1987) Psychiatric consultation liaison nursing and psychiatric nursing doctoring: similarities and differences. *Archives of Psychiatric Nursing*, 1 (2): 73–80.

Robinson, R.G., Bolla Wilson, K., Kaplan, E., Lipsey, J.R. & Price, T.R. (1986) Depression influences intellectual impairment in stroke patients. *British Journal of Psychiatry*, 148: 541–547.

Rogers, P., Curran, J. & Gournay, K. (2004) The person with an anxiety disorder, In: I. Norman & I. Ryrie (eds) *The Art and Science of Mental Health Nursing*. Maidenhead: Open University Press.

Roper, N., Logan, W. & Tierney, A. (2000) *The Roper–Logan–Tierney Model of Nursing*. Edinburgh: Churchill Livingstone.

Royal College of Physicians/Royal College of Psychiatrists (1995) *The Psychological Care of Medical Patients: recognition of need and service provision*. London: The Royal College of Physicians Publication Unit.

Royal College of Psychiatrists (1996) *Psychiatric Services to Accident and Emergency Departments* (Council Report 43) London: RCPsych.

Royal College of Psychiatrists/Royal College of Physicians/British Medical Association (2001) *Stigmatisation Within the Medical Profession. (Council Report 91)*. London: RCPsych.

Royle, J.A. & Walsh, M. (1992) *Watson's Medical Surgical Nursing and Related Physiology*, 4th edn. London: Baillière Tindall.

Russell, P. (2002) Social behaviour and professional interactions. In: R. Hogston & P.M. Simpson (eds) *Foundations of Nursing Practice*. Basingstoke: Palgrave Macmillan.

Ryrie, I. & Norman, I. (2004) Assessment and care planning. In: I. Norman & I. Ryrie (eds) *The Art and Science of Mental Health Nursing*. Maidenhead: Open University Press.

Sartorius, N. (1998) Stigma: what can psychiatrists do about it? *The Lancet*, 352: 1058–1059.

Savage, J. (1995) *Nursing Intimacy: an ethnographic approach to nurse–patient interaction*. London: Scutari Press.

Sharpe, M. & Peveler, R. (1996) Deliberate self-harm, substance misuse and eating disorders. In: E. Guthrie & F. Creed (eds) *Seminars in Liaison Psychiatry*. London: Gaskell.

Simpson, M., Buckman, R. & Stewart, M. (1991) Doctor–patient communication: the Toronto statement. *British Medical Journal*, 303: 1385–1387.

Smith, L.D. (2000) The nature of health and the effects of disorder. In: T. Thompson & P. Mathias (eds) *Lyttle's Mental Health & Disorder*, 3rd edn., pp. 21–30. London: Ballière Tindall.

Smith, P. (1992) *The Emotional Labour of Nursing*. Basingstoke: Macmillan.

Steinhausen, H.C. (2002) The outcome of anorexia nervosa in the 20th century. *American Journal of Psychiatry*, 159: 1284–1293.

Storer, A. (2000) The accident and emergency department. In: *Liaison Psychiatry: planning services for specialist settings*. London: Gaskell.

Stuart, G.W. (2001) Anxiety responses and anxiety disorders. In: G.W. Stuart & M.T. Laraia (eds) *Principles and Practice of Psychiatric Nursing*. St Louis: Mosby.

Sundeen, S.J., Stuart, G.W. & Ranking, E.A.D. (1998) *Nurse–client Interaction*. St Louis: Mosby.

Turp, M. (2001) *Psychosomatic Health*. Basingstoke: Palgrave Macmillan.

United Kingdom Central Council for Nursing, Midwifery and Health Visiting (1999) *Fitness for Practice*. London: UKCC.

Warner, R. (1994) *Recovery from Schizophrenia: psychiatry and political economy*. London: Routledge.

Wessely, S., Rose, S. & Bisson, J. (2000) Brief psychological interventions ('Debriefing') for trauma related symptoms and the prevention of PTSD. Cochrane Database of Systematic Reviews (2) P: CD000560.

White, R. (1985) *The Effects of the NHS on the Nursing Profession 1948–1961*. London: King's Fund.

World Health Organization (2003) *International Classification of Diseases and Related Health Problems 10*. Geneva: WHO.

Zigmond, A.S. & Snaith, R.P. (1983) The Hospital Anxiety and Depression Scale. *Acta Psychiatrica Scandinavica*, 67: 361–370.

Websites

Department of Health website: www.dh.gov.uk
National Statistics website: www.statistics.gov.uk

Chapter 2
Psychological Responses
to Illness and Injury

Chapter aims

This chapter will:

- describe the philosophical influences on professional perceptions of health and illness
- identify the role played by personal health beliefs on an individual's perception of illness and injury
- identify the various coping styles that may be adopted by those recovering from illness and injury, and during recovery and rehabilitation
- describe the process of psychological adaptation following illness and injury
- identify the essential components of effective psychological care.

Introduction

There is no 'normal' or routine response to the experience of illness, injury, hospitalisation or recovery. Each person is likely to experience a range of emotional reactions to being unwell, or to the circumstances of attending hospital or accessing health care, as it is a unique event. Therefore, the responses and reactions cannot necessarily be predicted. That said, it is possible to appreciate the various types of emotional, behavioural and interpersonal responses that a person may go through, or communicate to others as a result of becoming unwell. In order to understand these it is necessary to:

- appreciate the impact of the individual's health and illness beliefs in informing their responses to being unwell
- attempt to develop an understanding of them as an individual and the unique impact that current events may be having upon factors such as their ability to communicate and their individual behaviour

- be aware that there is no such thing as a 'normal' or 'abnormal' response to the experience of illness or injury
- assess and plan care that pays attention to the person as a unique individual.

Influences upon health and ill health

Western biomedical thinking is dominated by the belief that illness and disease can be reduced to a set of symptoms, which in turn leads to diagnosis of a specific illness or recognition of a particular disease process. In its broadest sense this is known as 'the medical model', and is a defined way of thinking about and explaining disease on the basis of biological factors (Barry & Yuill, 2002).

The biomedical perspective developed following the Enlightenment, a period from the late seventeenth century onwards, which was characterised by the advance of scientific knowledge, most notably developments in the understanding of anatomy and physiology, primarily as a result of examining the body post-mortem. This enabled doctors to understand the anatomical and physiological disturbances that occurred in certain diseases, whereas prior to this point, the factors that influenced people's understanding of illness included religion, spiritual beliefs, planetary movements, the activity of spirits, and even witchcraft (Hayes, 2000). The former perspective developed into what became known as a 'rational' explanation of disease, in that it is based on logical thinking and physical examination. Until this point, thinking about health and illness had been influenced by early Greek, Hebrew and Egyptian philosophies, which maintained that the mind and body were inextricably linked. Prior to the Enlightenment, therefore, notions of health and illness were essentially holistic in nature.

The other major influence in the development of biomedicine was the theories of the French philosopher René Descartes, who developed the idea that the mind and body were two separate and distinct entities. Descartes' view was that because the body is a material object it can be understood by scientific study and physical examination. He believed that the mind, however, is of a higher order and can therefore only be understood through introspection. This perspective separates the mind and body into two entities and so is dualistic in nature (Turp, 2001). A dualistic perspective considers an illness to be either somatic (physical) or psychic (mental) in origin. Both these theoretical perspectives paved the way for the development of what we now understand as biomedicine, with its emphasis on a linear cause-and-effect explanation of illness, the presence of observable symptoms and the reduction of the person's health problem(s) to the physical workings of the body (Barry & Yuill, 2002). This is in contrast to Eastern philosophies, which make no such distinction between a person's physical and mental states (Turp, 2001).

It is important to appreciate the impact that biomedicine has had, not only on our understanding of health and illness, but also upon how it informs the planning, organisation and delivery of health care (Eysenck, 1995).

Contemporary heath services are often separated according to whether they are primarily there to deliver physical or mental health care, thus providing a structural barrier to the practice of holistic care provision. Nursing training and education has traditionally mirrored this demarcation, with the separation of pre-registration adult (largely physically orientated care) and mental health branches.

Although in the latter half of the twentieth century there was an increasing emphasis by both doctors and nurses on the psychosocial determinants and impacts of illness, fundamentally, the biomedical perspective continues to dominate both our understanding of health and illness, as well as the way in which health care services are organised and delivered. Theorists have stressed how important the concept of holism is to nursing, yet much nursing practice continues to be delivered from a biomedical or dualistic perspective, as opposed to one that understands and embraces the bio-psycho-social needs of the person requiring care (Edwards, 2001). Such a gap between theory and practice is nowhere more apparent than in the general hospital where nurses are required to address the person's psychological needs against the backdrop of a system and service designed to treat and care for physical health problems as a discrete entity.

Thus it can be seen that a number of structural factors may militate against the provision of holistic nursing care. Such boundaries are firmly established and awareness by individual nurses of the need to practise from a holistic perspective may not always be enough to ensure that equal attention is paid to the person's physical and emotional needs. The development and use of nursing models within physical care settings, which provide a theoretical framework upon which to base nursing practice, have also been criticised for their apparent tokenistic approach to holism and over-emphasis on the physical aspects of care (Tierney, 1998; Walsh, 1998).

Personal beliefs, understandings and interpretations of health and illness

Becoming unwell is a stressful experience and one that will affect each person in a unique way. The impact of being unwell or of being admitted to hospital will be influenced by a wide variety of different factors (Fig. 2.1). The degree to which each factor will impact on the individual will be influenced by their:

- beliefs about health and ill health
- degree to which he or she feels 'in control' of what is happening to them
- current interpersonal, social and spiritual context
- repertoire of personal coping skills or techniques
- way in which he or she has responded to or dealt with stressful situations and life events in the past.

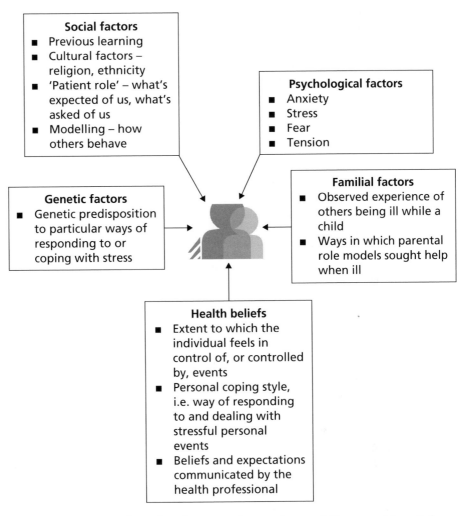

Social factors
- Previous learning
- Cultural factors – religion, ethnicity
- 'Patient role' – what's expected of us, what's asked of us
- Modelling – how others behave

Psychological factors
- Anxiety
- Stress
- Fear
- Tension

Genetic factors
- Genetic predisposition to particular ways of responding to or coping with stress

Familial factors
- Observed experience of others being ill while a child
- Ways in which parental role models sought help when ill

Health beliefs
- Extent to which the individual feels in control of, or controlled by, events
- Personal coping style, i.e. way of responding to and dealing with stressful personal events
- Beliefs and expectations communicated by the health professional

Figure 2.1 Factors influencing the person's experience of illness and hospital admission.

Health beliefs play an important role in the way in which the individual is likely to respond to the experience of being unwell, yet it is often the case that many health care staff do not always appreciate and acknowledge the unique and sometimes idiosyncratic health beliefs of individual patients (Maben & Macleod-Clark, 1995).

Most patients will perceive the experience of being unwell as a stressful event. Stressful events in relation to health care are often those that are perceived as new, unpredictable and uncontrollable, and will often involve a degree of change and loss. The impact of the illness is significantly influenced by the person's perception of the illness and their interpretation of what it may mean, as much as the illness itself (Rotter, 1966).

The person's interpretation of their illness will also be influenced by their personal coping style, as well as the degree to which they feel in control of what is happening. Some individuals will cope with their illness by limiting the amount of information they receive, and this may be demonstrated by behaviours such as not asking questions, or avoiding discussion of the implications or effects of their illness or injury. Others may deal with their experience by actively seeking out information or repeatedly requesting reassurance and explanations from staff.

Becoming unwell is often a frightening and a usually unwanted intrusion into the individual's life. Patients are likely to experience a sense that they

Table 2.1 Locus of control and its impact on health, illness and recovery.

Perspective	Description	Possible impact on illness and recovery
Internal health locus of control	People who view health, illness and recovery as being determined and influenced by their own behaviour and actions	More likely to take personal responsibility for their health and wellbeing View themselves as working in collaboration with the health professional to overcome health problems More likely to assimilate health promotion messages and to act on these, e.g. adopting a healthier lifestyle to prevent illness or aid recovery
External health locus of control	Individuals who view health, illness and recovery as something that has occurred or happens to them as a result of external factors	Likely to demonstrate a passive and reactive response to being unwell Unlikely to take the initiative in determining how he or she will overcome or deal with their health deficits or problems
Fatalistic perspective	A further example of an external locus of control, with the person believing that their illness and recovery will be largely influenced by factors such as fate, luck, or as an inevitability	Likely to demonstrate a fatalistic view of what has happened or is likely to happen to them May appear indifferent towards health promotion information or advice given by health professionals May not implement changes in lifestyle designed to reduce risk, as he or she believes that such changes are unlikely to make a difference May demonstrate this type of belief system with statements such as, 'Well, it's got to happen to someone' Unlikely to take responsibility for initiating strategies to promote or enhance recovery

Based on Grady & Wallston, 1990; Sarafino, 1994.

have lost control due to the enforced alterations and adjustments that may have to be made to their life. A further influence on health, the concept of ill health, recovery and coping, is the theoretical concept known as 'health locus of control theory' (Grady & Wallston, 1990; Sarafino, 1994). Health locus of control theory identifies three different determinants as exerting an influence on health and ill health, which are known as the internal locus of control, the external locus of control and the fatalistic perspective (Table 2.1).

Understanding the person's individual locus of control can help the professional to appreciate what may be behind certain behaviours and can also provide a basis for determining how much or what type of information the person may require about their illness. Although the health locus of control theory is helpful in understanding an individual's beliefs, this is only one perspective that needs to be considered when caring for individuals who have been ill or have experienced an injury. In practice, there is a complex interplay of various psychological, social, historical and interpersonal factors that will influence how the person responds, copes and adapts to being unwell (Wilkinson, 1999).

Coping and adaptation to illness and injury

The process of coping with hospitalisation, illness, recovery and being unwell involves a number of factors that can be described as the coping process (Moos, 1984). These consist of:

- thinking about the illness, injury or diagnosis
- identifying ways in which to cope with, respond to or deal with the problem
- planning and implementing particular strategies and responses.

Figure 2.2 provides a diagrammatic overview of the coping process. Hospitalisation, illness and feeling unwell are all life events that will involve a degree of stress, and to cope with this stress, the person will invoke a range of personal 'coping strategies'. The strategies employed will be influenced by a variety of other factors, in particular the repertoire of coping skills or methods that the person normally uses when faced with stressful situations. These coping strategies can be divided into those that are problem focused and those that are emotion focused (Baum *et al.*, 1997), although as stated above, which strategy is employed will vary from person to person and individual reactions may involve strategies from each group (Box 2.1). It is important to be aware that a person is unlikely to adopt just one or two methods of coping, but that they may use a range of strategies as they move through the experience of being unwell, or as their health needs change or develop as rehabilitation and recovery progress. The choice of coping strategy is unlikely to be a conscious one, and it is important to be aware of this when making suggestions to a patient about new or additional ways of coping. Some responses, however, may be considered less desirable than those identified above and can include:

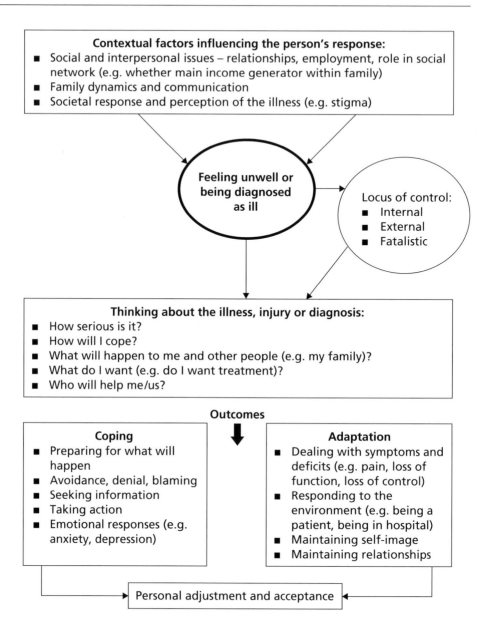

Figure 2.2 The process of coping with being unwell (based on Ogden, 1996).

- Denial – This may involve ignoring or denying symptoms, sometimes to the extent that the person delays seeking help. It can also influence the degree to which the health professional achieves concordance regarding treatment decisions (e.g. taking medication) and co-operation with nursing care.
- Unrealistically hoping that the condition will go away or resolve of its own accord.

> **Box 2.1** Range of possible coping strategies people may adopt as a result of becoming unwell.
>
> Problem-focused
>
> - Seeking out information and advice from staff, peers, family and friends
> - Actively looking to develop new skills, e.g. yoga, relaxation techniques
> - Seeking practical and social support, e.g. joining a local support group or service user forum
> - Developing new or additional interests as a direct result of the illness experience, e.g. joining Friends of the Hospital
> - Active participation in treatment and care decisions, e.g. requesting updates or clinical reviews from medical staff, making suggestions regarding new or alternative treatment options
> - Helping others
>
> Emotion-focused
>
> - Expressing anger, frustration or other distressing feelings, e.g. crying
> - Talking about and sharing feelings with others
> - Acknowledging and recognising loss
> - Seeking emotional support from new or alternative sources, e.g. attending church or other religious meetings, joining a support group
> - Adopting a realistic perspective regarding prognosis and recovery, e.g. may be demonstrated by making plans for the future that involve not being part of the individual's current network
> - Becoming emotionally distant or disconnected, e.g. temporarily shutting off and focusing on other tasks or problems

- Excessive focusing on specific symptoms or deficits caused by the illness, to the extent that recovery and rehabilitation is adversely affected.
- Seeking to apportion blame to someone or something else when there is no legitimate reason for doing so.

Adapting to an illness or diagnosis is a dynamic process and will be influenced by any or all of the factors identified above. It can sometimes be tempting for health professionals to focus exclusively on the illness or disability, without paying adequate attention to the individual's personal history, background, relationships, personal context and coping style. This can be observed when staff make statements such as 'Well, he's had a stroke, so he would be depressed, wouldn't he?'. Although changes in mood and emotional lability are common experiences following an illness such as a stroke, it is important that it does not detract from the ability of staff to see such responses as unique to the individual. Always expecting and accepting that a person will become depressed may mean that significant pathology and distressing symptoms may be overlooked and treatment inadvertently withheld (Mumma, 1986; Bennett, 1996).

Table 2.2 Model of adjustment.

Stage	Indicated by
Initial impact	Shock and denial
Defence mobilisation – implementation of psychological defences	Bargaining Denial Minimising the seriousness or importance of the situation
Initial realisation	Mourning Depression Internalised anger
Retaliation and rebellion	Anger and aggression are externalised, e.g. projecting feelings of anger onto partner or other family member
Reintegration and reorganisation	Acknowledgement Acceptance Final readjustment Reconstruction and rebuilding life and relationships

Adapted from Livneh, 1986.

Livneh (1986) likens the psychological events following a major illness or disability to the grieving process. Individuals will usually experience shock and disbelief, denial, depression, grief, anger and acceptance, although not necessarily in that particular order (Table 2.2). For example, in the initial period following a diagnosis, denial may act as a protective mechanism, shielding the person emotionally from the overwhelming nature of what they have been told.

Acute stress reactions

In recent years the term 'post-traumatic stress' has been used to describe the range of emotional and physical reactions that an individual might experience following a significant traumatic event. Such events can include the experience of a major illness or injury, particularly if it has occurred suddenly and has ongoing lifestyle and adjustment implications. The prevalence of post-traumatic stress disorder (PTSD) is approximately 1% in the general population, and although the condition has been recognised as a consequence of acute illness, research studies have largely focused on rates in survivors of specific types of trauma, such as bomb survivors, rape survivors and those who have experienced the sudden unexpected death of a loved one (Rogers & Liness, 1999).

Within the general hospital it is more likely that individuals will demonstrate signs and experience the symptoms of an acute stress reaction (ASR). An ASR can occur following any experience of illness, trauma or injury, although as with PTSD it is more likely when the events have occurred suddenly and appear to be outside the individual's control. It is important to appreciate that it is not necessary for the person concerned to have been physically involved in the trauma; witnessing a traumatic event can be enough to trigger an ASR. For example, the patient who witnesses the sudden collapse of a fellow patient, has to call for help and then either observes or hears the frantic attempts of staff to resuscitate the person.

Acute stress reactions are usually self-limiting and in most cases do not require any specific physical treatments, such as medication. However, the symptoms can be severe and distressing for the individual and may include the following:

- Vivid visual and auditory recall of the events or trauma – 'flashbacks'
- Excessive tiredness
- Jumpiness and an exaggerated startle response
- Dizziness
- Tearfulness
- Palpitations
- Mood swings
- Nausea
- Feeling shaky
- Shortness of breath in the absence of physical exertion
- Headaches
- Non-specific muscular pains
- Persistent fear that the traumatic event will re-occur
- Loss of interest in sex.

The above symptoms can occur within a few hours and are likely to be at their most severe in the first two weeks following the trauma. If marked symptoms persist in their frequency and severity for longer than four weeks, then the condition will need to be re-classified as PTSD (Rogers & Liness, 1999).

Explanation, information and reassurance are essential elements of a nursing care plan for the person experiencing an ASR, and staff should consider the appropriateness of supplying the individual with written information as an adjunct to verbal explanations. Normalising the experience can be of value, as is reassuring the person that he or she is not 'going mad'. Involvement of significant others and the family is also important, as they are likely to notice a number of psychological and behavioural changes in the person as a result of the original trauma.

Impact of illness on families and carers

High rates of depression have been identified in individuals caring for a person with a physical illness (Krishnasamy *et al.*, 2001). Whether it is chronic and ongoing or short lived, any illness or disorder may be viewed as an 'unexpected guest' who needs to be incorporated into the family and its relationships for the duration of their stay. Family members' initial expectation of whether it is likely to cause death, along with the experience of anticipatory loss, are crucial factors to the outcome of chronic illness (Rowland, 1990). To master the challenges of chronic conditions, individuals, couples and families usually need to re-negotiate the rules and roles in their relationships and aim to incorporate the sometimes unfamiliar dynamics of the patient–caretaker relationship. For example, when a woman is diagnosed as having breast cancer, open communication between her and her partner is one of the most important components in maintaining the secure relationship needed to cope with the illness (Dale & Altschuler, 1999).

However, communication between people will vary and is largely determined by established interpersonal communication patterns that have developed over years and possibly decades. Important discussions for couples, families and carers may consist of gathering information about the illness or condition, as well as coping with the biological, psychological and social demands that may result. Human nature often means that people are concerned and curious about things such as:

- how the illness or condition came about
- whether they did anything to cause it
- whether they could have done anything to prevent it
- whether it is contagious or can be inherited.

The nurse has a role in supporting and guiding the patient and family through their quest for knowledge and understanding about the illness and possible consequences. In certain instances, particularly with terminal illnesses, discussions about wills, specific family arrangements and advance directives may be important. An important message to convey in certain situations is that couples and families can, and do, learn to use the awareness that all relationships are time limited. With this in mind it can be possible to live life more fully in the present and enjoy what they have in the 'here and now' rather than postpone fulfilment based on an illusion of infinite time (Rowland, 1999).

The involvement of significant others with treatment therefore becomes even more important; however, time and resources will determine the ability to involve family members in the patient's treatment while in hospital. Whenever possible, nursing staff should actively involve the person's significant other(s) in the planning and delivery of care and, with the patient's agreement, in the planning of treatment decisions and preparation for discharge, rehabilitation or death. This means that it is important to do more than simply keep family members informed of the patient's progress or be available to answer specific questions. Each family situation and dynamic will vary, but, if achievable, good practice should be that the partner or family member is included in discussions on a regular basis. In some circumstances, an individual patient may request that other members of his family are not informed of specific details regarding the care or treatment programme, and these wishes must be respected. However, such requests for non-discussion with family members can in themselves provide a useful therapeutic platform upon which to explore with the patient his fears, anxieties and concerns regarding the sharing of information within the family. As with many forms of 'bad news', the reality may be that other members of the family are already aware of the seriousness of the person's condition, or of the fact that they have limited time left as a family unit or as a couple. In such circumstances it may be more appropriate to view the practitioner's role as acting as a facilitator for effective communication, rather than the bearer of bad news *per se* (see Chapter 5).

Nursing priorities in the provision of psychological care

In order to provide effective psychological care, it is important to address this in a structured way. As described above, patient reactions and responses to their situations will vary, although certain nursing actions are required to ensure that a person's psychological needs are responded to effectively. Psychological care requires that practitioners:

- are aware of verbal and non-verbal communication, e.g. making good eye contact, tone of voice, body posture
- pay attention and use active listening when talking with the person, e.g. avoid excessive note taking during an interview or conversation
- use open-ended questions, e.g. 'In what way has this problem affected you?', as a means of encouraging expression and clarifying problems
- make empathic comments, e.g. 'This seems to be a really difficult time for you'
- respond to verbal and non–verbal cues, e.g. if the person becomes restless when discussing a particular subject, it may be appropriate to pick up on this, 'You seem to find it uncomfortable when we talk about your relationship'
- pay attention to contextual, relationship and family issues, e.g. elicit what has been the person's history and experience of illness and treatment within the family; ask how family members view the problem and how the current problem is affecting other members of the family, e.g. children
- identify the person's unique concerns – these may be relatively straightforward to deal with, but paradoxically can cause an inordinate amount of distress, e.g. How will the person's partner get to hospital to visit them if he or she cannot drive?

As with all other aspects of the individual's care and treatment, psychological care should be approached and delivered systematically. It can be tempting to minimise the need for both psychological care and support, as well as the role of the practitioner in providing it. Statements such as 'We talk to the patient when we're giving a bed bath', or 'It's OK to sit down and talk to patients once we've done all the work' are both examples of how psychological care is de-valued when compared with more tangible examples of the nursing role, and of how it is often seen as an additional nicety, as opposed to a vital aspect of good clinical care.

Gask and Underwood (2003) identify three essential components of good psychological care:

(1) *Providing information.* Review the amount of information you provide – is it the right amount, at the right time and concerning the right issues? Traditionally we have provided information based on what we think the person needs to know or should know, but information needs to be provided in a way and at a time that is driven by the patient (Nichols, 2003). If adequate attention is paid to the provision of information, it can act as a form of reassurance and emotional support, as well as reduce anxiety. The impact of cognitive impairment, the person's cultural and ethnic context, and any sensory or learning difficulties also need to be taken into account when providing information (Kessels, 2003).

(2) *Negotiating a care plan.* This is a dynamic process and every attempt should be made actively to involve the patient in the development of an individual plan of care. This will include ascertaining expectations, responding to requests for information and advice on particular treatment or care options, developing and documenting what will happen and what the patient can expect. As during the assessment phase, it is necessary to 'think family' and include their role and input into specific areas of the treatment and care plan. While paying attention to the individual's underlying health beliefs, coping style and degree of adjustment, it is important to check his or her understanding of what will happen next. Consider too the use of a brief written summary for both the patient and their family.

(3) *Appropriate use of reassurance.* Providing reassurance is often identified as a significant role for the practitioner, but is only useful if you know exactly what it is the person is anxious, concerned or worried about. Simply reminding the person that 'Everything will be all right', or that 'There's nothing to worry about', are likely to increase levels of anxiety, rather than reduce them. Arbitrarily limiting the amount of information provided is also more likely to have the opposite effect, '"the less they know, the less they worry", is a dangerous myth' (Nichols, 2003).

Dealing with emotions

The process of adjustment and coping may involve a range of emotional reactions, some of which may leave the practitioner uncertain about how to respond. Such emotions can include denial, anger, fear, tearfulness and anxiety, and the person may present with these in what appears to be a chaotic manner. As has been discussed, these responses should be viewed as a 'normal' reaction to the situation that the patient finds himself or herself in. On some occasions, emotional outbursts may be triggered by apparently minor events or problems and will be compounded by factors such as tiredness, exhaustion and feelings of isolation and powerlessness. It is therefore just as important to offer help with these underlying problems, while at the same time remaining calm and acknowledging the impact that both the emotional and the practical factors have had on the person's mental state.

Overt displays of emotional distress can be difficult for some staff to cope with and, in an attempt to minimise their own distress, they may seek to avoid discussion of the underlying issue and move on to matters that are less distressing. However, in order to provide effective psychological care, practitioners need to be able to react with confidence and calmness, responding to the emotional cues and using these as an opportunity to explore the underlying difficulty or anxiety.

Denial

Many individuals will appear to deny the fact that they are unwell, or to appear overly optimistic in the face of a poor or terminal prognosis. Denial is a common reaction to hearing devastating news and should be seen as part of the overall process of adjustment and coping. It is usually transitory in nature and is often apparent at the start of an illness or upon having a diagnosis confirmed. Psychologically, denial often acts as an unconscious defence mechanism, whereby it provides a way of limiting and dealing with the overwhelming emotions that patients find themselves experiencing.

It is important not to attempt to force the person into acknowledging or accepting the situation, diagnosis or prognosis. Denial should not be seen as a 'problem' in itself, but rather as a metaphor or strategy for dealing with painful emotional material. It may in fact be more appropriate to help the person address the fears or anxieties that underlie the denial. How it is addressed will also be influenced by the kind of support that is available to the patient and by their current interpersonal and family situation.

Anger

Becoming angry can also act as an emotional protection as the person struggles to come to terms with their situation or diagnosis. Being angry can be a temporary way of shifting the focus from the individual and how they might cope, on to other things. When dealing with a person who is verbally angry, it is important to avoid a defensive response or to act in a similarly hostile way. Acknowledging the underlying feelings, and providing the person with an opportunity to discuss these further in a supportive and caring environment is a useful strategy. If the person or their family have specific concerns or complaints, staff should ensure that these are taken seriously and should indicate that the required action will be taken to ensure that these are either investigated or dealt with.

Fear

The things that trigger a perception of fear will be unique to each individual. Some patients may harbour unrealistic fears concerning their diagnosis or prognosis, for example, fearing that a diagnosis of cancer will inevitably be terminal, or that all treatments for the disease will cause hair loss. It is important to address what it is the person fears, providing relevant information and explanation at regular intervals. New or additional fears may develop as the person's illness or treatment progresses, so it will be necessary to review this on a regular basis.

Tearfulness

Becoming tearful is a universal experience and is often the outward manifestation of painful or pent-up emotional material. It is important to acknowledge this and recognise that many people will find crying a cathartic and restorative experience. Staff should not ignore someone who is tearful or crying, but use it as an opportunity to demonstrate empathy with his or her underlying distress and as a chance to engage in a supportive conversation. While crying can be a sign of marked internal distress, and as such requires a response from those nearby, it is also a way of releasing suppressed and pent-up emotions. In some situations it can be entirely appropriate to provide the person with the time and emotional space to cry in privacy and without repeated interruptions.

Anxiety

Anxious reactions are common in people who are facing uncertainty about their situation as a result of illness. The process of attending at or being admitted to hospital, with its unfamiliar environment and strange routines, can also be a source of considerable anxiety. Anxiety can manifest in a variety of ways, including an increased sense of panic, unease and apprehension, along with being irritable, impatient and agitated. Anxiety will also reduce the person's tolerance to pain and increase levels of physical discomfort and muscular tension. Other common symptoms of anxiety include palpitations, breathlessness, loss of appetite, insomnia and tightness in the chest. In certain illnesses, such as acute cardiac events, the patient may misinterpret these symptoms as being signs of an exacerbation of their coronary condition. This in turn can lead to a vicious cycle of anxiety and further chest pain, necessitating additional investigations and resulting in delays to recovery and rehabilitation.

A number of strategies and interventions can be useful in helping the anxious person. Providing information about anxiety is important, and this may be enough to reassure and reduce its impact in some people. Other people, however, may require more specific interventions, such as developing relaxation techniques, learning how to undertake breathing exercises and diversional activities, such as taking a warm bath, talking, engaging in a practical task or having a warm drink.

Conclusions

Psychological responses to illness and injury are influenced by a series of complex interactions involving the person's social, interpersonal and cultural background, and their beliefs about health, illness and the experience of recovery. Set reactions cannot be predicated and each person will present with a unique range of responses. In order to ensure that people who have experienced illness, injury and hospitalisation have their care delivered in a holistic way, it is necessary for practitioners to develop an understanding of the theoretical perspectives behind the psychological responses to illness and injury and to ensure that this informs the development of care planning and nursing interventions aimed at ensuring effective psychological care.

Nurses have a unique role in helping to bridge the gap between the physical and psychological elements of care by ensuring that they have a depth of understanding that allows them to address the issues discussed in this chapter. More detailed exploration of these issues and the improved appreciation of the psychological impact of illness and injury will ensure that as a professional group nurses develop the professional confidence to reclaim this important aspect of care.

References

Barry, A. & Yuill, C. (2002) *Understanding Health*. London: Sage Publications.

Baum, S., Newman, S. & Weinman, J. (1997) *Cambridge Textbook of Psychology, Health and Medicine*. Cambridge: Cambridge University Press.

Bennett, B. (1996) How nurses in a stroke rehabilitation unit attempt to meet the psychological needs of patients who become depressed following stroke. *Journal of Advanced Nursing*, 23 (2): 314–321.

Dale, B. & Altschuler, J. (1999) In sickness and in health: the development of alternative discourses for families with parental illness. *Journal of Family Therapy*, 21: 267–283.

Edwards, S.D. (2001) *Philosophy of Nursing*. Basingstoke: Palgrave.

Eysenck, H.J. (1995) Mental health and physical disease: a new paradigm. *Journal of Mental Health*, 4: 221–225.

Gask, L. & Underwood, T. (2003) The consultation. In: R. Mayou, M. Sharpe & A. Carson (eds) *The ABC of Psychological Medicine*, pp. 1–3. London: BMJ Books.

Grady, K.L. & Wallston, B.S. (1990) *Research in Health Care Settings*. Newbury Park: Sage.

Hayes, N. (2000) *Foundations of Psychology*. London: Thompson Learning.

Kessels, R.P.C. (2003) Patients' memory for medical information. *Journal of the Royal Society of Medicine*, 96: 219–222.

Krishnasamy, M., Wilkie, E. & Haviland, J. (2001) Lung cancer health care needs assessment: patients' and informal carers' responses to national mail questionnaire survey. *Palliative Medicine*, 15: 213–227.

Livneh, H. (1986) A unified approach to existing models of adaptation to disability: a model of adaptation. *Journal of Applied Rehabilitation Counselling*, 17 (6): 5–16.

Maben, J. & Macleod-Clark, J. (1995) Health promotion: a concept analysis. *Journal of Advanced Nursing*, 22: 1158–1165.

Moos, R.H. (1984) *Coping With Physical Illness: new perspectives*. New York: Plenum Press.

Mumma, C.M. (1986) Perceived loss following stroke. *Rehabilitation Nursing*, 11 (3): 19–24.

Nichols, K. (2003) *Psychological Care for Ill and Injured People*. Maidenhead: Open University Press.

Ogden, J. (1996) *Health Psychology*. Buckingham: Open University Press.

Rogers, P. & Liness, S. (1999) Post-traumatic stress disorder: nature, assessment and psychological treatment. *Mental Health Practice*, 2 (5): 29–37.

Rotter, J. (1966) Generalised expectancies for internal vs external control of reinforcement. *Psychological Monographs*, 80 (1): 1–26.

Rowland, J.S. (1999) Anticipatory loss: a family systems developmental framework. *Family Process*, 29: 229–244.

Sarafino, E. (1994) *Health Psychology: biopsychosocial interactions*, 2nd edn. New York: John Wiley.

Tierney, A.J. (1998) Nursing models: extant or extinct? *Journal of Advanced Nursing*, 28 (1): 77–85.

Turp, M. (2001) *Psychosomatic Health*. Basingstoke: Palgrave.

Walsh, M. (1998) *Models and Critical Pathways in Clinical Nursing*. London: Baillière Tindall.

Ward, B. (1999) Improving the detection of postnatal depression. *Professional Nurse*, 15 (1): 15–18.

Wilkinson, J.A. (1999) Understanding patients' health beliefs. *Professional Nurse*, 14 (5): 320–322.

Chapter 3
The Legal and Ethical Context of Mental Health Care in the General Hospital

Chapter aims

> ## This chapter will:
>
> - identify the key legal, ethical and professional principles in relation to the provision of mental health care within the general hospital
> - discuss the concepts of capacity, competence, consent and duty of care as they relate to the general hospital
> - discuss the use and application of the Mental Health Act 1983 within the general hospital.

Introduction

The legal and ethical principles that underpin nursing practice may, at times, appear complex in relation to caring for people with mental health problems in the general hospital. Anecdotal evidence suggests that this is an area of practice that many nurses find challenging, as well as one that can cause high levels of professional anxiety. Staff practising in the general hospital may also feel that they lack knowledge regarding the legal principles that pertain to a person who is experiencing mental health difficulties. Added to this is the seemingly complex issue of the application of the Mental Health Act 1983 within the general hospital, and the tensions generated by the various ethical, legal and professional expectations of the nurse.

This chapter will identify the key ethical, legal and professional perspectives that need to be considered when caring for a person with mental health problems in the general hospital. Examples used in this chapter pertain to current English statute and case laws, as applicable to England and Wales. Different statute law applies to both Scotland and Northern Ireland, although

Table 3.1 Characteristics of statute and common law.

Statute law	Common law
Usually drafted by the Government; its relevance and enactment is openly debated in the UK or European Parliament prior to becoming law	Also referred to as case law or judge-made law
The law is written down and it can be consulted and referred to by others	These are laws based on the decisions made by judges in individual cases. The 'Bolam principle' is an example of case law informing health care practice, when the case of Bolam v Friern Hospital Management Committee (1957) produced a definition of what is reasonable in terms of the standard of competence expected of health staff carrying out their duties
Statute laws take precedence over all other laws	
Statute law is applicable as long as it remains on the statute – the only way for legislation to cease to be law is for it to be repealed	They may be based on interpretations of statute law (but not necessarily so), or as a result of cases brought before a panel of judges by individuals or organisations such as NHS trusts
Examples of statute laws relevant to health care include the Health and Social Care (Community Health and Standards) Act 2003, Nurses, Midwives and Health Visitors Act 1997, Mental Health Act 1983 and the Mental Capacity Act 2005	A further example of common law principles applied to health care is the concept of a 'duty of care'. The fact that health professionals and NHS trusts owe their patients a duty of care has been established in common law (Dimond, 2002)

the majority of the general principles (specifically those relating to ethical practice and professional conduct) outlined here are equally applicable to the whole of the UK.

The terms 'Statute Law' and 'Common Law' will be referred to throughout, and it is therefore important that there is clarity regarding these principles. Statue law refers to laws that can be called the 'laws of the land' (Table 3.1).

The ethical and professional context

A nurse's practice is informed and governed by a variety of factors, all of which reflect her unique role in the care and treatment of patients. Factors that guide and inform professional practice include:

■ *Legal requirements.* For example, the need to be on a register of nurses before practising as a registered nurse; the need to maintain professional competence to fulfil a duty of care owed to the patient (Dimond, 2002). Other legal requirements, in particular specific statute laws, also inform

Table 3.2 Examples of statue laws directly applicable to nursing.

Statute	Comments
Mental Health Act 1983	Allows for the compulsory detention and enforced treatment for mental illness and disorder Nurses need to be aware of the common 'sections' of the act and its relevance to their area of practice (Knowles, 2003)
Access to Health Records Act 1990	Allows individuals to access their health (including nursing) records (Grange, 1998)
Human Rights Act 1998	Enshrined in law are the following rights (Persaud & Hewitt, 2001): 　The right to life 　The prohibition of torture and inhuman and degrading treatment 　The right to liberty 　The right to respect for private and family life 　Freedom of expression 　The prohibition of discrimination
Freedom of Information Act 2000	Gives the right to access written information from public bodies (including health care providers) The type of information that can be requested must be the type that will not cause significant harm, for example, to national security or the ability to enforce the law. Members of the public may request information relating to NHS trust policies, e.g. local policy on the prescribing and administration of medication
Mental Capacity Act 2005	Sets out the legal terms under which it is possible to make decisions – including those relating to health care – for people who are not able to make decisions for themselves

how nurses practise and need to be adhered to during our contact with patients and their relatives (Table 3.2).

■ *Ethical requirements.* The need to respect the right of the individual to make decisions about their care (autonomy); the need to avoid inflicting harm (non-maleficence); the need to do good (beneficence); the need to treat people fairly and with respect (justice) – (Beauchamp & Childress, 1994). Implicit within this ethical framework is the need to avoid paternalism, whereby health care professionals assume that they always know what is best for the patient. While their motivation may be informed by the desire to do good, this always needs to be balanced with the individual's right to autonomy.

■ *Professional requirements.* The obligations laid down in the *Code of Professional Conduct* (Nursing and Midwifery Council, 2002). The code requires that the nurse acts at all times in the best interests of the patient, meaning that all actions and omissions will be measured against this standard. Although this code is not legally binding, failure to act within its boundaries would constitute a breach of the code and can provide evidence of failure to follow approved practice (Dimond, 2002).

The nature of mental illness, the presentation of acute distress and the impact of behavioural disturbance can present specific challenges to nursing and other health care staff within the general hospital. Not every individual will behave in a characteristic or stereotypical way, that is, by being co-operative, compliant, uncomplaining and grateful. Numerous factors will influence the way in which people respond to the experience of being unwell or in hospital, many of which will be underpinned by feelings of acute fear, stress and anxiety, sometimes leading to difficult or challenging behaviour (see Chapters 2 and 4). On occasion, such difficulties may manifest by the patient refusing to consent to treatment, lacking the capacity to make decisions, or refusing to accept well intentioned advice or requests from staff. Examples may include the person with marked cognitive impairment, the person with an acute exacerbation of a mental illness, and the individual who is profoundly depressed and expresses a wish to be allowed to die. In these circumstances it is necessary to reflect on the ethical framework that informs nursing practice.

Since the 1980s there has been an increasing awareness of the need to ensure that health care and nursing are delivered in a way that is acceptable to those who use our services. The development of the service user movement within mental health services has occurred against a backdrop of the recognition that it is not acceptable for patients or families to be cast in the role of passive recipients of treatment and care. However, ensuring meaningful involvement of patients and carers in their care requires health staff to practise from a sound ethical-driven perspective. Shifts in professional attitudes, from paternalism (the professional knows best) to respect for the person's autonomy (the patient decides), require nurses to address real-life ethical issues on a daily basis (Young & Fawcett, 2002).

The individual's right to autonomy is held to be one of the fundamental principles of sound ethical practice. However, in reality, respecting the person's right to exercise their own free will can produce major dilemmas for health care staff. In denying a patient who is expressing suicidal ideas the right to leave hospital without further assessment and treatment, the nurse concerned needs to ensure that the seriousness of the harm that might befall the patient is of such a magnitude that it warrants limiting autonomy (Lauder *et al.*, 2005). Intervention in such a situation is based on utilitarian ethical philosophy espoused by Mill (1963) and known as the 'harm principle'. Adhering to the harm principle means that a degree of intervention that limits a person's autonomy may be justified in such a situation. The same principle is being followed when the state enacts legislation that limits individual autonomy in order to reduce the likelihood of harm to the rest of society. Examples of such interventionist policies aimed at minimising harm include the legal requirement to wear seatbelts in cars and the ban on smoking in public places.

Ethical decision-making does not occur in a vacuum, but is informed by a complex interplay of professional judgements, ethical principles and legal requirements. Reconciling all these factors within the health care setting can be challenging, and nurses should ensure that they seek the appropriate level of advice, support and supervision to enable them to participate in decision-making that is based on sound ethical principles. As a result, all treatment and nursing care needs to be informed and planned within the relevant ethical, legal and professional frameworks, and this includes the need to keep up to date and achieve competence when providing care to individuals experiencing mental health problems and psychiatric illness.

The legal context: decision-making, capacity and competence

An understanding of the concepts of capacity and consent are vital in order to ensure that the patient's autonomy and right to self-determination are respected. Common law in England and Wales recognises that all adults have the right to refuse any treatment that is offered to them, as long as they possess the capacity to make such a decision (Re C, 1994). It does not matter why the person is refusing the proposed treatment, or even whether the choice is rational or irrational, or whether it is clear why the person has made such a choice (Bellhouse *et al.*, 2001). This legal right remains even if the likely outcome is detrimental to the person concerned. However, this right to self-determination is only meaningful and of value as long as the person has been adequately informed, has the mental ability to make a decision and has been free to make the decision without coercion (Grisso, 1986). Individuals who decide to refuse treatment can pose a significant challenge for the health care team, as the person's wishes may be in direct contrast to those of the staff or others, including relatives or next-of-kin.

It is necessary to understand the terms 'capacity' and 'competence' as applied to the health care setting (Box 3.1), as it is these principles that ensure the nurse is able to determine whether a person has given valid consent for a treatment or investigation to be carried out. Being clear about whether a person possessed the capacity to make a decision is also important because health staff are coming under increasing pressure to demonstrate how they reached a decision regarding a person's competence (Wingfield, 2003).

When in hospital, certain individuals may lack competence to make decisions regarding their health care or about proposed treatments and this is termed incapacity (Bellhouse *et al.*, 2001). Incapacity may be permanent or temporary, for instance, someone who is intoxicated after drinking a large amount of alcohol will temporarily lack capacity, although a person who has sustained serious brain damage as a result of a head injury is likely to suffer from a

> **Box 3.1** Understanding capacity and competence.
>
> ■ In England and Wales there is no legal definition of capacity, although the Law Commission (1995) have defined a person as lacking capacity if they are 'unable by reason of mental disability to make a decision on the matter in question, [or they are] unable to communicate a choice on that matter because he or she is unconscious or for any other reason'
> ■ The terms 'capacity' and 'competence' are usually used interchangeably, although competence is the clinical equivalent of the legal concept of capacity (Tan & Elphick, 2002)
> ■ Capacity and competence are concerned with the mental ability of a person to make a decision
> ■ An adult is assumed to have competence unless it can be proved otherwise
> ■ Competence must not be confused with the professional's assessment of the reasonableness of the person's decision

permanent lack of capacity. There are a number of other causes of incapacity, some of which may be temporary, including:

■ General anaesthesia
■ Delirium
■ Shock
■ Intoxification – from alcohol, drugs, etc.
■ Sedation
■ Dementia
■ Learning disability
■ Mental illness – the presence of a mental illness does not necessarily mean that the person lacks capacity, although this may be the case as a result of some psychiatric illnesses. Case law has established that the person with a mental illness may still be deemed competent to make decisions regarding treatment (Re C, 1994). The only way to establish whether the person lacks capacity is to apply the test of competence.

To determine whether a person has capacity and is competent to consent to treatment, they must:

■ understand the information being given to them, especially in relation to the consequences of having or not having the intervention in question
■ retain the information
■ use and weigh up that information in their decision-making process.

In England and Wales, the concept of capacity has formed part of common law jurisdiction and until 2005 was not defined by statute. The Mental Capacity Act 2005 has formalised previous common law principles, identifying a framework for assessing capacity, with built-in legal safeguards to protect patients (Irons, 2004). In Scotland incapacity is enshrined in law as a result of the Adults with Incapacity (Scotland) Act 2000. As with common law, the provisions of this act assume that the individual has the capacity to make their own decisions unless it can be proved otherwise. This act contains specific provision for the administration of medical (and nursing) treatment to an adult who is unable to give consent.

Consent

The concept of consent is derived from the ethical principle of autonomy, and informed consent respects the person's right to autonomous self-determination (Booth, 2002). In practice, there are three distinct types of consent:

(1) *Written consent.* This is represented by a signed document from the patient confirming that they have given their consent to the proposed intervention.
(2) *Verbal consent.* The patient verbally gives consent by saying 'Yes'.
(3) *Implied consent.* There is no written or verbal agreement, but the person indicates their willingness to go ahead with the proposed intervention by their behaviour and physical gestures, for example, proffering an arm to the nurse when she explains that she would like to obtain a blood sample.

All three forms of consent are equally valid (Department of Health (DoH) 2001a) although in practice, written and verbal consent should be obtained for all potentially serious investigations or interventions, for example, surgical procedures and general anaesthesia. Where there is disagreement or the proposed treatment has been challenged, then it is important to document the decision-making processes and rationale for the proposed treatment, as well as obtaining specific written consent (British Medical Association, 2002).

There is no legal process whereby another person (including the individual's next-of-kin or nearest relative) can consent to something on behalf of the patient (DoH, 2001b). While it is good practice to involve the person's partner, family or significant other in treatment and care planning, it is not possible for any of these individuals to provide consent, and the professional has a duty to act in the patient's best interests (Re F, 1990). If the person lacks capacity, then the wishes of family members should be taken into account when reaching decisions about treatment and on-going care, but the eventual outcome will be the responsibility of the practitioner, based on their assessment of what is in the patient's best interests. The legal context regarding capacity and consent is clear, although recently the issue of whether people with illnesses that cause permanent incapacity are unable to give consent has been challenged, with calls to ensure that decisions regarding capacity are informed not only by the legal definitions, but also by factors such as personal wellbeing, personhood, previously stated wishes, beliefs and preferences (Dewing, 2001).

> **Box 3.2** Information required to make an informed decision.
>
> To make a health care decision the individual must understand in broad terms:
>
> - The nature of the proposed intervention
> - The purpose of the proposed intervention
> - The risks and benefits of the proposed intervention
> - The possible risks associated with not carrying out the proposed intervention
> - The possible risks and benefits of alternative interventions

For consent to be valid it needs to be given voluntarily and the patient must be in possession of all the relevant information pertinent to the intervention being proposed (Box 3.2). Consent is not necessarily valid just because the patient has signed a consent form; it is up to the practitioner to demonstrate that they provided the information required for informed decision-making.

The *Code of Conduct* provides guidance in relation to consent and refusal to treatment, stating

> *'When patients . . . are no longer legally competent and thus have lost the capacity to consent or refuse treatment and care, you should try to find out whether they have previously indicated preferences in an advanced statement. You must respect any refusal of treatment or care when they were legally competent, provided that the decision is clearly applicable in the present circumstances and there is no reason to believe that they have changed their minds'* (Nursing and Midwifery Council, 2002).

Duty of care

Nurses, by virtue of the nurse–patient relationship, owe their patients a duty of care and need to ensure that they do not come to any unnecessary harm as a result of negligence or omission (Dimond, 2002). Duty of care is established through common law and is applicable to all health care settings and individual professionals. By being accountable for their actions, nurses demonstrate the duty of care they owe to patients. Exercising a duty of care means that as an individual professional, the nurse must take responsibility for ensuring that she is competent to meet the care needs of her patients. NHS trusts and other institutions responsible for the organisation and provision of health services also have a corporate duty of care, and as such have to ensure that there are adequately trained staff and facilities to meet the needs of patients.

At times the individual practitioner's duty of care may appear to be in conflict with the patient's right to autonomy and self-determination. For example, it can be difficult to reconcile the wishes of an individual patient to refuse treatment (autonomy) with the professional and legal obligation to provide care. In essence the nurse needs to demonstrate that her actions were:

> **Box 3.3** Case study – patient's apparent expressed wishes versus the nurse's duty of care.
>
> Mark was brought into the emergency department by ambulance after falling over in the street and sustaining a deep laceration to his left arm. Mark was accompanied by two friends, who explained that he had consumed a large amount of alcohol earlier in the day. Mark smelt of alcohol, his speech was slurred, he was irritable and was staggering around the department. Nurse Hopkins, who was caring for him, explained that he would need to have an X-ray of his arm in order to ensure that no foreign bodies were present, prior to his wound being cleaned and sutured. Mark refused to have an X-ray, claiming that he was 'allergic to radiation', and instead wanted to go home. Due to his level of intoxication, Mark was temporarily unable to demonstrate that he had capacity to make an informed decision. Nurse Hopkins and the hospital trust owed Mark a duty of care, however difficult or unco-operative he may have been. To have allowed him to go home without the X-ray may well have been negligent. As a result, Nurse Hopkins asked Mark's friends to remain with him at the hospital until the worst effects of the alcohol had worn off. Two hours later, Mark approached Nurse Hopkins, apologised for his earlier behaviour and agreed to undergo an X-ray of his arm.

- reasonable
- in the patient's best interests
- undertaken with the patient's informed consent.

The exception to this would be when the person fails the test of capacity – in this case, the practitioner's duty of care will need to inform subsequent nursing actions. In the example in Box 3.3, the situation was managed effectively by postponing a decision until the patient had regained capacity.

An important principle in deciding whether to act contrary to a patient's expressed wishes concerns the issue of 'reasonableness', which means to what extent the practitioner can directly intervene in a particular situation or with a particular patient. For example, if a person is admitted following a deliberate overdose of medication, it would be reasonable to ask the patient whether he had any substances on his person that he could harm himself with while in hospital. It is reasonable because we know the risks associated with overdose and that a number of people are likely to repeat their actions (see Chapter 8), even while in hospital. To ask the question of the patient demonstrates accountability to our duty of care and can be considered a reasonable thing to do, illustrating our commitment to patient safety. However, despite being aware of the potential risk of repeat self-harm, it would be unreasonable in this situation to search the patient and his personal belongings without his permission, as the degree of force used in this action would be disproportionate to the degree of risk posed.

The principle of acting contrary to a patient's expressed wishes (or in the absence of knowing whether they would wish you to proceed) is connected to our duty of care as professionals. Common law provides the legal framework by which medical and nursing staff can:

- detain someone against their will
- give urgent treatment to someone who lacks capacity to give consent.

In practice, common law allows an individual to apprehend or restrain a person if there are reasonable grounds to believe that person poses a significant danger to themselves or others and would continue to do so if allowed to leave. The degree of physical intervention, such as physical restraint, should be enough to bring the emergency situation to an end, but no more. Any restraint that involves excessive force, or which continues after the immediate crisis is over, is not justified. The fundamental issue here is an assessment of the person's capacity to make a decision.

In order to ensure that the most appropriate actions are taken and that staff act in the patient's best interests, it is necessary to consider all the relevant factors and events that have led to the current situation; this will include issues such as the person's previously expressed wishes, views of family and significant others, and an evaluation of the risks and benefits of intervening versus not intervening (Wingfield, 2003). A framework for reflecting in practice is suggested in Table 3.3 as a means of planning actions in situations that may be challenging or complex (Harrison, 1997).

Table 3.3 Framework for responding to patients who lack capacity.

Consider	Rationale
Patient safety – does the person present an immediate risk to himself or others?	If refusing the proposed intervention is likely to have life-threatening consequences for the patient or others, then intervention is justified under common law If failing to act is subsequently proved to have been negligent, then the practitioner will be in breach of her duty of care

Do you possess all the relevant information about the situation?	It is important to obtain as much collateral history and supporting information as possible. Sources of information will include:
	    The person's family or significant other
	    Background to the current presentation
	    Current social or interpersonal difficulties/problems
	    Effects of alcohol or illicit drugs on the person's mental state
	    Effects of shock, sedation or medication on the person's ability to communicate
	    The person's previously expressed wishes regarding the situation, e.g. have they prepared an advanced directive regarding treatment in this situation?

Table 3.3 (*Cont'd*)

Consider	Rationale
Your knowledge and skills base – do you consider yourself confident to respond to this situation?	Ensure that you and your colleagues have adequate training and access to clinical supervision All registered practitioners should be competent in the assessment of capacity (Ball & Macdonald, 2002) Ensure that the unit or department has up-to-date policies and clinical guidelines in place for the management of such situations, e.g. do you know how to access specialist help, are you aware of your role as a registered nurse in assessing capacity, what support and advice can you expect to receive, e.g. additional staff, access to on site security personnel? See Chapter 8 for additional information

What alternatives are available to you in this situation?	If the situation is not life-threatening, then it may be possible to plan alternatives to direct physical intervention
	Wingfield (2003) suggests the following should be considered:
	  If safe to do so, postponing the decision about intervention until capacity returns
	  Securing as much involvement of the person as possible, even if he lacks full capacity
	  Involving others, such as family or close friends in the decision-making process and the delivery of care. Those who know the person well may be very skilled at reducing the individual's level of arousal and agitation
	  Taking the least restrictive option available at the time

Use of the Mental Health Act (MHA)	The MHA only allows for treatment of a mental illness, not a physical illness or treatment of the physical consequences of a mental illness. Therefore it is of little use in the immediate management of challenging or complex situations Although a registered medical practitioner can apply to detain a person using the MHA (Section 5[2]) for up to 72 hours, this cannot be used within the emergency department, as it only applies to those patients who are admitted to the hospital. If it is considered that restraint or forcible treatment is needed in the patient's best interests, then this action will need to take place under the umbrella of common law
Consequences of not acting	You need to be able to defend and justify your actions should the need arise. It is therefore important to ensure that the rationale for the course of action chosen is clearly described and documented in the patient's record. Details of conversations with family, relatives and colleagues also need to be recorded

The Mental Health Act 1983

The essential function of the Mental Health Act (MHA) is the protection of individual patients, as it provides explicit detail of what health and social care professionals are authorised to do in relation to the detention and enforced treatment of those suffering from a mental illness. The present act came into effect in 1983 and operates on a prophetic rather than historic basis, being the only item of peacetime legislation that allows an individual to be detained against their will, for long periods of time, on the basis of what clinicians think that that individual might do, rather than on what they have already done (Melia *et al.*, 1999). The MHA is designed for the treatment of mental illness and mental disorder, not physical illness or the physical consequences of a mental illness. This means that treatment (including nursing interventions) without consent for anything other than a mental illness would constitute battery and is an offence (Bellhouse *et al.*, 2001).

There is, however, an exception to the above rule, which applies in the case of individuals suffering from anorexia nervosa. Because of the inextricable link between physical and mental symptoms in severe anorexia nervosa, physical treatment, such as forced re-feeding, is considered lawful under the provisions of the MHA (Mental Health Act Commission, 1997). As highlighted elsewhere in this book, individuals with mental health problems may experience co-morbid or coincidental physical ill health that requires admission to the general hospital (see Chapter 10). As a result, there will be occasions when clinical staff may be called upon to make an application for a detention under the MHA, and to provide care to individuals who are already subject to a detention under the act.

The MHA is interpreted for practitioners, mainly doctors, nurses and social workers, through the *Mental Health Act Code of Practice* (DoH and Welsh Office, 1999) and provides detailed guidance on its use, and all practitioners, including those in the general hospital, who may be likely to care for a person who is subject to the provisions of the MHA should have ready access to a copy. The act referred to here is applicable only in England and Wales; separate mental health legislation applies to Scotland and Northern Ireland.

The MHA is divided into ten parts or sections, which is where the term 'sectioning' comes from. Not all sections of the act are of direct relevance to the general hospital, although a number of sections are seen in this setting with some frequency (Table 3.4). It is important to remember that it is not the doctor who 'sections' a patient, but the hospital managers who detain the person on the medical recommendation of the doctor (or appropriately registered nurse).

The application of the MHA can be a complex and time consuming process, particularly for staff who do not have to deal with it on a frequent basis. However, it is important to remember that failure to ensure that the act is interpreted accurately or to ensure that patients are only detained as specified

Table 3.4 Sections of the Mental Health Act 1983 that are commonly encountered in the general hospital.

Section	Duration of detention	Reason	Comments
2	Up to 28 days	Assessment	Generally used if the person has no recent history of admission under the act, or where the diagnosis is unclear. The patient has the right of appeal to the hospital managers and a Mental Health Review Tribunal within 14 days of admission
3	Up to six months	Treatment	It is unlikely that section 3 would be applied within a general hospital. Patients subject to section 3 are likely to already be receiving treatment under the Act in an inpatient mental health unit, but may be transferred to a general hospital ward for treatment of a physical illness
5(2)	72 hours	Detention of a person who is already receiving voluntary inpatient care	This is the section most likely to be used within a general hospital. It is also known as the 'doctor's holding power', as its purpose is to trigger a full assessment under the act. The patient's Responsible Medical Officer (RMO) must make the application to the hospital managers using the appropriate documentation. This task can be delegated to a more junior doctor, excluding pre-registration house officers. The patient is not detained under the act until the hospital managers have received and accepted the relevant papers. Treatment without consent (except any that needs to be given as a life-saving measure) cannot be given while the patient is subject to section 5(2)
136	72 hours	Detain a person who a police officer suspects to be suffering from a mental illness	Like Section 5(2), this is a holding power that triggers a full assessment under the act. The person detained must be taken to a 'place of safety'*, usually a police station or a hospital. There is no formal documentation that accompanies this section, although individual police authorities will have their own administrative arrangements in place

* Place of Safety is not defined in law, but is a matter for local determination. The relevant NHS trust, police force and local authority must all agree as to where the local place of safety is. Good practice is that the place of safety should not routinely be the local police station (custody suite), but rather an appropriate health care setting.

in the legislation, will result in the person being detained unlawfully. In such circumstances, the patient may have a case against the individual practitioner or health trust for unlawful detention or breach of human rights (Persaud & Hewitt, 2001). The Mental Health Act Commission (2004) provides detailed guidance for general hospitals in the application of the MHA. A number of common problems occur when the act is applied within the general hospital and include:

- *Incorrect reason for detention.* The MHA only allows for detention and treatment relating to a mental illness, so for example, citing the need to give physical treatment for an overdose (such as intravenous medication) is not allowed.
- *Enforcing physical treatment to a non-consenting patient.* Treatment can only be given against a person's expressed wish in certain circumstances.
- *Failing to ensure that the relevant MHA documentation has been accepted by the hospital managers.* Unless this takes place, the detention is invalid.
- *Failing to provide the patient and his or her nearest relative with written and verbal information regarding their rights.* Under the MHA, patients have certain rights, for example, to speak with an advocate and access legal representation; therefore, it is essential that these rights are explained in easy-to-understand language.

Conclusions

This chapter summarised the relevant ethical, legal and professional requirements of the nurse in relation to the care of people with mental health problems in the general hospital. A heavy emphasis was placed on the importance of nurses developing clarity regarding the relevant legal frameworks that have to inform care planning and delivery. In particular, an understanding of informed capacity, informed consent and duty of care is vital if nurses are to provide care that is legally and professionally defensible. However, providing care that meets legal requirements is but one dimension, and all practitioners need to ensure that a sound ethical framework guides their relationships and interventions for patients and their families.

References

Ball, C. & Macdonald, A. (2002) Clinical capacity assessment. *Psychiatric Bulletin*, 26: 394.

Beauchamp, T. & Childress, J. (1994) *Principles of Biomedical Ethics*, 4th edn. Oxford: Oxford University Press.

Bellhouse, J., Holland, A. & Clare, I. (2001) Decision-making capacity in adults: its assessment in clinical practice. *Advances in Psychiatric Treatment*, 7: 294–301.

Booth, S. (2002) A philosophical analysis of informed consent. *Nursing Standard*, 16 (39): 43–46.

British Medical Association (2002) *Consent Toolkit*. London: BMA.

Department of Health (2001a) *Reference Guide to Consent for Examination or Treatment*. London: Department of Health.

Department of Health (2001b) *12 Key Points on Consent: the law in England*. London: Department of Health.

Department of Health and Welsh Office (1999) *Mental Health Act 1983 Code of Practice*. London: The Stationery Office.

Dewing, J. (2001) Older people with mental illness and administration of medicines: consent and capacity. *Mental Health Practice*, 5 (4): 33–38.

Dimond, B. (2002) *Legal Aspects of Nursing*, 3rd edn. London: Pearson Longman.

Grange, A. (1998) Patients' rights to access their healthcare records. *Nursing Standard*, 13 (6): 41–42.

Grisso, T. (1986) *Evaluating Competencies: forensic assessments and instruments*. New York: Plenum.

Harrison, A. (1997) Consent and common law. *Nursing Times*, 93 (52): 52–54.

Knowles, J. (2003) Care and treatment under the Mental Health Act 1983. *Nursing Times*, 99 (19): 30–32.

Irons, A. (2004) Living wills – the dilemma. *New Law Journal*, June: 966–967.

Lauder, W., Davidson, G. & Anderson, I. (2005) Self-neglect: the role of judgements and applied ethics. *Nursing Standard*, 19 (18): 45–51.

Law Commission (1995) *Mental Incapacity: a summary of the Law Commission's recommendations*. London: HMSO.

Melia, P., Moran, A. & Mason, T. (1999) Triumvirate nursing for personality disordered patients: crossing the boundaries safely. *Journal of Psychiatric and Mental Health Nursing*, 6: 15–20.

Mental Health Act Commission (1997) *Guidance on the Treatment of Anorexia Nervosa under the Mental Health Act 1983*. (Guidance Note 3), Nottingham: MHAC.

Mental Health Act Commission (2004) *Use of the Mental Health Act 1983 in General Hospitals without a Psychiatric Unit*. Nottingham: MHAC. See www.mhac.trent.nhs.uk

Mill, J. (1963) *Collected Works of John Stuart Mill*. Toronto: University of Toronto Press.

Nursing and Midwifery Council (2002) *Code of Professional Conduct*. London: NMC.

Persaud, A. & Hewitt, D. (2001) European convention on human rights: effects on psychiatric care. *Nursing Standard*, 15 (44): 33–37.

Re C (*Adult: Refusal of Medical Treatment*) (1994) 1 All ER 819.

Re F (*Mental Patient: Sterilisation*) (1990) 2 AC 1.

Tan, J. & Elphick, M. (2002) Competency and use of the Mental Health Act – a matrix to aid decision-making. *Psychiatric Bulletin*, 26: 104–106.

Wingfield, J. (2003) Consent and decision-making for patients who lack capacity: what should pharmacists know? *The Pharmaceutical Journal*, 271: 463–464.

Young, J. & Fawcett, T. (2002) Artificial nutrition in older people with dementia: moral and ethical dilemmas. *Nursing Older People*, 14 (5): 19–21.

Chapter 4
Caring for the Person Displaying Challenging Behaviour

Chapter aims

This chapter will:

- explore the nature of challenging behaviours
- outline the most common causes and triggers of disturbed behaviour
- outline the process of risk assessment
- describe a range of management strategies and approaches to deal with challenging behaviour.

Introduction

Caring for patients who present a 'challenge' in some form or another is part of the emotional labour integral to nursing. The ability to be caring does not come naturally, but it is something nurses have to develop within themselves emotionally, irrespective of their personal feelings, about themselves, their patients, or the conditions and circumstances in which they work (Smith, 1992). In so doing, nurses learn to manage their emotions more effectively and 'manage' challenging situations and patients more positively[1] – something that has always been a core part of nursing. Difficulties in the nurse–patient relationship can be traced back beyond the advent of 'modern' nursing in the mid-nineteenth century. However, it is only in recent years that serious

---

[1] We have used the term challenging behaviours because it reminds us that people are not intrinsically challenging; it is about the relationship between the person 'challenging' and the person feeling challenged. However, much of the literature still concerns the 'difficult patient' and, as such, we will use this term in discussion.

debate about the subject has taken place. This is partly because nursing is now more closely regulated than ever, and issues of public protection have come to the fore. At the same time, there has been growing concern regarding the numbers of assaults on nurses (and other health workers), abuse, violence and the impact on nurses in terms of stress and time away from work. Concepts such as 'zero tolerance' have gained common currency, and government targets have been established and training programmes to deal with the issue have been implemented.

This chapter explores the nature of challenging behaviour, attempting to offer a new perspective on familiar terms such as 'the difficult patient' and 'manipulative behaviour'. In discussing the causes and triggers of challenging behaviour, it examines not only the individual nurse–patient relationship but the context in which it occurs, highlighting the external factors that impact upon the behaviour of both parties. It also explores how nursing responses – or the lack of a response – can lead to behaviours which then challenge the practitioner. Risk assessment and safe strategies for managing challenging behaviours are obviously vital but this chapter will also detail more pro-active methods of both understanding and addressing the issue. The need to care for people who exhibit challenging behaviours will always be an issue for nurses and nursing, and this chapter hopefully suggests clear strategies for responding to it and minimising the negative impact that it can have.

The nature of challenging behaviours

There is a fundamental belief that goes back at least as far as the Old Testament story of Jonah. It is that all would be well 'if only the evil ones, the trouble makers, could be got rid of' (Obholzer & Roberts, 1994). Nursing has its own version of this which translates – only half in jest – into something like, 'Nursing would be very easy – if it wasn't for the patients'. Yet, for many years, it was difficult for any nurse to admit she was finding it difficult to 'cope' with the demands of either the work generally or the impact of a particular patient. Perhaps this is one of the reasons why the topic of challenging behaviours features so little in the nursing literature, despite voluminous writings on the nurse–patient relationship, most of which speak of 'unconditional acceptance' and 'empathic understanding', without necessarily acknowledging or addressing the difficulty these can pose for a nurse trying to care for a patient she finds particularly challenging.

The point of Obholzer and Roberts' (1994) observation was to claim that, in some respects, we have a need for someone who is 'difficult' or 'challenging'. This argument suggests that those who are 'troublesome' are, in fact, 'unconsciously selected by the institution' for the wider purpose of helping us feel better about ourselves, being blamed for all our difficulties, meaning the responsibility does not lie with us. Indeed, the phenomenon of a 'difficult patient' should be regarded as a symptom of, and not as a disturbance to,

Table 4.1 Examples of behaviours that can be experienced as challenging.

Complaints	Class discrimination
'Splitting' (see Fig. 4.1)	Silence and/or withdrawal
Non-adherence with investigations or treatment	Avoidance or denial
The patient who does not improve – this might be in the form of someone whose pain cannot be controlled or the patient who presents a new set of symptoms as soon as a previous set of symptoms has resolved	Dependence, which can manifest through constantly demanding attention from staff or an insatiable desire to be noticed
	Anxiety and distress
Sexual disinhibition	Confusion
Sexism	Self-harm
Racism	Grief
Non-co-operation	'Being ill'

clinical work. The most obvious kinds of challenging behaviour, in the form of violence or aggression, either verbal or physical, can be overt and obvious. However, it can assume a variety of more subtle forms (Table 4.1).

Individuals are often identified as 'difficult' within the first 24 hours of coming into hospital (Ritvo, 1963), if not before they arrive on the ward, and this form of labelling can have a detrimental effect on the patient. However, it is more than the attribution of a label; it is a process, growing out of the individual's interaction with significant others (in this case, nurses and other health care professionals), their expectation of him and his behaviour (Slevin, 2003). It can lead to stigmatising and stereotyping, prompting discrimination from the dominant group and disengagement by the individual.

So-called difficult patients have also been attributed certain key characteristics, including emotional instability, high levels of anxiety, depression, hostility and being overtly dependent or independent, aggressive, unappreciative, non-conforming and manipulative (Ritvo, 1963). 'Manipulative' behaviour is one of the most commonly described behaviours that nurses find difficult, and it is usually interpreted as being motivated by the patient's conscious intention to gain a particular response from the nurse (Gatward, 1997). Although it is often so transparent that it is greeted with anger and/or rejection, those who feel they have been subjected to attempts at manipulation, successful or otherwise, often react with a sense of having been, at best, used or, at worst, abused.

The actual meaning of the term manipulate is, 'Handle; deal skilfully with; manage craftily' (Coulson & Carr, 1976). Of course, it is the lack of skill displayed by most 'difficult' patients that is their problem. The ability to handle, deal with and manage relationships is crucial to their success, whether personal or business. Dexter and Walsh (1995) suggested the use of the word 'orchestrative' to define this behaviour. When a nurse feels something as powerful as having been manipulated or abused after any interaction, it can be helpful to understand that this may be the only way the patient can communicate his own affect, or feeling, projecting it through the behaviour (Casement, 1986). Thus, were the patient able to articulate his feelings, they would very often be similar to those the nurse feels after the interaction of being confronted with a particular behaviour. Sundeen *et al.* (1998) described projection as:

> *'A defence mechanism that occurs when the feelings, wishes, or attitudes of the person are attributed by him to another person (or object). The person feels that it is unacceptable to have these impulses. He seeks to place blame for his inadequacies on someone else; this other person is thought to be responsible for causing his mental anguish.'*

An example of this may occur when a patient continually criticises nurses for not being 'good enough', when, actually, *he* feels that he is not good enough. Ridley (1993) suggests that animals use communication less for transferring information than to manipulate one another. People are not really very different. Human communication is a complex set of negotiations, emotional trade-offs and manipulations rather than a simplistic mechanical exchange of information. Perhaps the real problem that challenging patients have is that they are not manipulative enough, or that their attempts are so regressed as to alienate the recipient of their attention (Linehan, 1993).

So it is with 'splitting', another common behaviour that often challenges nurses and ward colleagues. Splitting is a mental defence mechanism. As with all mental defence mechanisms, it is something anyone might employ, particularly when stressed or feeling vulnerable – as they may well do if they feel physically unwell or are facing uncertainty about their diagnosis and/or prognosis. Equally, the less well developed the individual, emotionally and psychologically, the more likely they will be to use mental defence mechanisms in a maladaptive way.

At its simplest level, splitting may manifest itself through a patient asking different members of staff for the same thing until he gets what he wants – particularly in a situation where the team has made a decision it expects everyone to stick with consistently. Additionally, the patient may then complain that the team is so disorganised that 'everyone' gives him a different answer. The individual may view people and situations as either all good or all bad when, in reality, it is almost always a mixture of both. This reflects an inability to integrate the positive and negative qualities of oneself (Stuart, 2001) (Fig. 4.1). In this context, the behaviours and communication of the patient and Nurse B are negative, reinforcing all the patient's worst feelings about himself. At the same time, the behaviours and communications of the patient and Nurse A are far more positive. The nurses then replicate the patient's own internal 'split' in their own discussion and enact his internal conflicts as they cannot agree about his behaviour and health care needs.

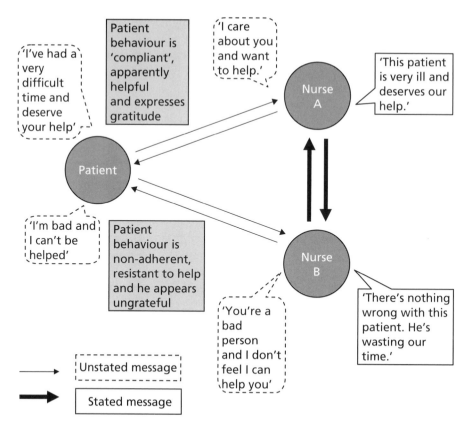

Figure 4.1 The patient with challenging behaviours: how maladaptive communication and splitting affect the patient-to-nurse and nurse-to-nurse relationships (adapted from Perlin, 2001). Note: Compliance is not the same as being adherent to, or in concordance with, treatment.

Breeze and Repper (1998) found that patients are identified as difficult when they pose a threat to the nurse's competence and control. Nurses define patients as difficult in a socially constructed manner, when the patient denies the authority and therapeutic value of the nursing staff, 'not as a result of the "difficult" behaviour'. Where nurses are perceived to demonstrate respect, time, skilled care and a willingness to give patients some control and choice in their own care, feelings of anger can be reduced. This implies the roots of challenging behaviour lie in the protagonist feeling powerless. There is an obvious irony in this, as many nurses ascribe great power or control to individuals engaged in challenging behaviours, experiencing powerful emotional responses, saying such things as, 'He makes me feel like . . .'. Indeed, challenging behaviours often result in a struggle for control or a series of responses from nurses and colleagues that do not address the problem, but establish a conflictual relationship. These forms of response merely perpetuate the problem and increase levels of frustration, since all parties involved are likely to become dissatisfied with the way they interact and the outcome of the conflict (Salla, 2000). Indeed, feeling misunderstood, 'not heard' or ignored, the patient may feel compelled to act in an even more challenging manner. This can be further contrasted with the 'ideal' patient, who is trusting, agrees without resistance to all therapy and procedures, expresses gratitude and is open when questioned but says nothing if not asked. Importantly, he suits the work pattern of the staff and does not challenge their authority (Geisler, 1991).

Causes and triggers of disturbed behaviour

Although challenging behaviours may have their origins in psychological responses and the context of health care, it is important to give wider consideration to the problem. For example, such behaviour can have an organic cause. Aggression in an older person may be due to electrolyte imbalance, while an apparently intoxicated patient's challenging behaviour may have less to do with alcohol than a head injury – although if intoxication is the cause of challenging behaviours, this needs to be addressed while maintaining clear boundaries around the limits of acceptable behaviour.

Challenging behaviours associated with Alzheimer's disease and related dementias may include restlessness, pacing and wandering, repetitive calling or questioning. The individual may become emotionally labile, apathetic and experience disturbed sleep. However, even in a patient with a dementia, this in itself may not be the cause of the challenging behaviour. For example, the patient may be experiencing physical pain due to something such as a toothache; the side effects of medication can cause behavioural disturbance, including confusion and agitation (see Chapters, 2, 7 and 12 for further detail). The physical discomforts from being too hot or too cold, or needing to go to the toilet can also trigger disturbed behaviour. Dehydration can cause dizziness, headaches, dry skin, infection, cramps, constipation, urinary problems and increased confusion, all of which can result in disturbed behaviour.

However, if there is no organic cause and the patient is not intoxicated, the behaviour must be treated as a communication, even if the person is suffering from a psychotic illness. Nursing staff may not think they can respond effectively to the result of a patient's thought disorder or psychotic content, but they can respond to his affect, for example, he may be feeling threatened, frightened or anxious. Anger and aggression are a response to the same physiological sensations that prompt the fight or flight response; therefore, leaving a psychotic patient in an anxious or frightened state may lead to an escalation of behaviour as he tries to communicate his feelings.

Figure 4.2 illustrates such a communication process. An external stimulus is received and the individual tries to make sense of this. We immediately try to place this in a context but this is mediated by our own experience and

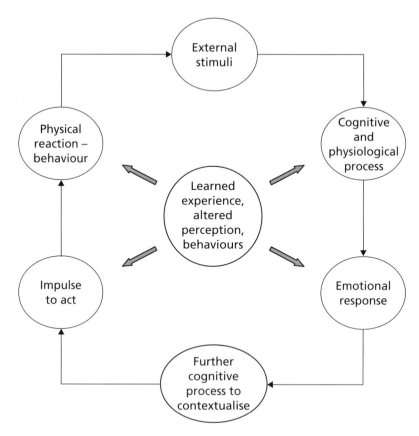

Figure 4.2 A model of communication for understanding challenging behaviours.

perception. The cognitive process overlaps with the emotional responses and the impulse to act is based on the judgement we arrive at. Examples are given in the case studies in Boxes 4.1 and 4.2.

The examples above illustrate how challenging behaviours can be used to communicate something the individual may be unable to articulate verbally. If this is the case, it is unlikely that he has any developed level of understanding about it and thus cannot communicate his emotional distress and/or disturbance in any other way. Given there are very few challenging patients, as opposed to people who present with challenging behaviour, a more objective criterion for assessing this can be achieved through undertaking a biographical history, which will provide some context to the person's current issues and problems. If a clear pattern emerges of, for example, difficulty in dealing with and responding to caring relationships, this will need to be taken into account. The person may be someone with a higher than usual, but well-founded, need for information or an inbuilt critical approach to problems. They may have grown into the role of a 'difficult patient' as a

Box 4.1 Case study 1.

An older man, suffering from a urinary tract infection, is being nursed in a four-bedded ward bay. He is pyrexial, nauseated and drowsy. It is his first night on the ward and he is slightly unsure of his whereabouts or the time. He is also missing his hearing aid. Dozing on his bed, he is woken by two nurses who want to take him to the toilet, as it stated in his nursing notes that he has problems with continence. It has been a very busy shift and they have a lot of tasks to complete. They take hold of his arms before he is properly awake. That is the external stimulus but, suddenly awoken, he cannot think what is going on. Adopting the fight or flight response, he tries to move away. The nurses, fearful he will fall, tighten their grip. He struggles free and pushes at one of the nurses. There is an angry exchange. The patient accuses them of 'doing things' to him but still feels slightly confused and cannot articulate his thoughts clearly. The nurses try to explain that he must not push them and that they were only trying to help. Unable to hear properly, but embarrassed and feeling this is yet another representation of his loss of independence, the patient falls silent and refuses to go to the toilet. Later, he has to urgently ask the nurse to bring him a urinal as he does not think he can get to the toilet in time. She is delayed and he is incontinent. He shouts at her and her response is that he could actually have gone to the toilet earlier in the evening.

The next time the two nurses approach the patient, he is immediately wary, withdraws and refuses to interact with them. In recording the incident, it is noted that he was 'confused and aggressive'.

Points for reflection:

- How could the nurses have handled this situation differently?
- What could they have said and done differently?
- In what ways has the information presented in this chapter so far enabled you to consider how you might interpret and manage similar types of behaviour in your own clinical setting?

result of experiences in which they received poor or disappointing treatment. Influences which are specific to the illness play a role, especially in chronic disease or prolonged and difficult hospitalisation (see Chapter 2).

What is it that challenges us?

Perhaps a good starting point when considering the patient's behaviour is to ask, who is it who finds it unpleasant, difficult or problematic? What is it about this person's behaviour that is difficult to manage specifically? From the patient's point of view, is it legitimate and understandable? We have already explored how the patient's psychological motivations and attempts to communicate might influence the outcome of such a question, although the nurse's own state of mind is equally important. Hantikainen (2001) notes

> **Box 4.2** Case study 2.
>
> Jane has been a patient on a haematology ward for several weeks, being treated for acute myeloblastic leukaemia and is being nursed in a single room. Initially chatty and cheerful, as her treatment with chemotherapy has progressed she has become more irritable, unwilling to have her observations recorded and even, on occasions, refusing treatments. She has also asked the nurses to stop visitors coming into her room.
>
> It emerges that, while having the treatment, she has been ruminating on her past, when she was psychologically and sexually abused by her father. He is now dead, but her mother is alive and Jane blames her mother for not being available to protect her when she was in need. Remembering this, she has re-experienced feelings of guilt and started having intrusive thoughts that she is not worth helping and, even if she were, the treatment will not be successful. She has begun to believe she is likely to die and then fears for her 2-year-old daughter's long-term welfare.
>
> She feels ashamed about her anxious and negative thoughts. She believes she has no control over them or the medical condition which has brought her into hospital, feeling her own body has 'turned against her'. Thinking that she has also lost control over what happens to her while in hospital she challenges the nursing staff at every opportunity.
>
> There is a series of confrontations between Jane and the frustrated nursing staff. It is only when a nurse from the mental health liaison team meets with her that she articulates these troubled thoughts and feelings. Jane then begins to be able to challenge both her feelings and the extremely negative image of herself that she has constructed. This enables her to become more relaxed about, and accepting of, her treatment regimen and negotiating her needs with the nurses.
>
> Point for reflection:
>
> - How could the nurses caring for Jane have avoided the cycle of frustration and confrontation?

there is often agreement among nurses on the use of negative labels such as 'difficult behaviour', which may even be communicated prior to contact with the patient and that:

> *'Behaviours that typically lead to the use of restraints [with older patients] have been described by nursing staff as disruptive, difficult, asocial, bizarre, deviant or inappropriate. A common denominator of all these labels is that the behaviour has been identified through interaction with others. It always appears as problematic in the environment. Nurses used restraints to exert an element of control over an otherwise chaotic situation, particularly if the behaviour was apparently irrational or inexplicable, and some behaviours were perceived as "an assault on their self-esteem and professional identity".'*

Reading these descriptors, it becomes apparent that there is a high degree of subjectivity, emphasising the interaction of nurse and patient in defining

Box 4.3 Case study 3.

Nurse Watson has almost finished a ten-hour shift in the emergency department (ED). Early in the shift, she was involved in a difficult interaction with a man who was extremely distressed by an accident involving his son. She had inadvertently given him some incorrect information and he had become very accusatory and critical. Later, she was involved in an unsuccessful attempt to resuscitate a car crash victim who was almost identical in age to her sister. Short of staff, the ED team had to cope with several angry outbursts and abusive behaviour from frustrated or intoxicated patients. Nurse Watson had planned to go to the library to get some books she needed for an essay which is almost overdue, but knows that the library has now closed. She is feeling angry and resentful at the way in which the demands of the job impinge on her life and, she feels, are holding her back.

A young woman who has been waiting to be seen, having presented to the department following a paracetamol overdose, comes out of her cubicle demanding to know where the doctor is. Tired and pre-occupied, Nurse Watson tells her she will have to wait. The young woman threatens to leave. Trying to talk to her about the implications of taking an overdose, Nurse Watson cannot articulate her thoughts clearly. The young woman starts shouting that the nurse knows nothing about her, her experience or anything at all. She tells Nurse Watson she is lazy and uncaring. Unable to respond and frightened that she will burst into tears, Nurse Watson leaves the area and avoids seeing the patient for the remainder of the shift. Having the next two days off, she replays the incident over and over in her mind, thinking of what the young woman said, feeling angry and resentful and unable to shake off those feelings. For the next week, she does all she can to avoid caring for both young women and people who have presented following self-harm.

Points for reflection:

- Why do you think this nurse had such difficulty in dealing effectively with the patient who had taken an overdose?
- What might have helped her to deal with her own feelings and professional frustrations?

'challenging' behaviours. What is asocial, or bizarre, or deviant? Indeed, what do we collectively mean by 'difficult'? Behaviours intolerable in one hospital or unit may be accepted in another. So the internal world of the nurse is as important as the behaviour itself. Moreover, what is challenging for a nurse on one day may have been manageable on another day. Why would it be challenging for one nurse but not her colleagues? So the question has to be broadened to consider what has been happening to the particular nurse – before an incident – that has made the event or behaviour so difficult.

Box 4.3 illustrates how everyday situations can challenge nurses, as well as identifying how communication with patients and families can inadvertently become challenging. Thinking once more of the model of communication and challenging behaviour (see Fig. 4.2), Case study 3 highlights the importance of the nurse's learned experience, perception and the context in which such difficulties arise, and that these factors clearly influence whether or not the nurse in question felt challenged. In this, the cumulative effect of a number of incidents that challenged her on different emotional and psychological levels, many not particularly conscious, finally takes its toll. Her reaction is against the last but, in some ways, the easiest. She feels unfairly offended and hurt. However, she was also carrying a variety of difficult feelings from her inter-action with the boy's father and felt very distressed during the unsuccessful resuscitation attempt, which had resonance for her regarding her sister. Finally, she is neither mindful of the young woman's needs nor able to formulate a helpful response to the patient's frustration, anxiety and anger, having recognised at some level that the woman was actually very worried about the potential effects of the paracetamol and still distressed by the events that led to her taking the tablets.

As has been noted above, challenging behaviour implies a threat, which evokes a defensive response. The perceived threat to one's self or self-image may be real or imagined. Brandon (1990) describes his difficulty with a student:

'I have taken to avoiding [her]. I feel she is bitter and angry in her dealings with me. Each time we meet I bring this belief and memory. I am hurt and respond angrily and dogmatically although I feel near to tears. My anger seems to feed her bitterness. I hardly see her. She becomes a walking symbol for the thousands of times that people seemed unkind and unjust.'

So it can be seen that conflict is inherent to challenging behaviours and, worse still, can be internalised. Conflict can be defined as the simultaneous presence of incompatible desires or goals (Sundeen *et al.*, 1998), and challenging behaviour causes conflict. This conflict may be 'acted-out', or displayed, by nurses avoiding certain patients, finding ways to retaliate, or challenging them in ways that only heighten their defences and reinforce their challenging behaviour. Alternatively, it can be addressed, and defused, although key to addressing it is answering the question: Is the patient's behaviour the problem, or our reaction to it?

The patient, the institution and the situation

A dysfunctional team or organisation is more likely to see an increase in the number of challenging situations. 'Zero tolerance' is now established in virtually every public service and no hospital corridor or ward notice board is complete without its poster warning that violence, verbal abuse or a range of behaviours towards staff will not be tolerated. It makes sense, of course. No one should have to come to work to be abused, threatened or, worse still, assaulted, yet Gournay (2002) found that 85% of nursing staff had experienced verbal abuse or been threatened with violence. But, as in any assessment, we have to ask the question, 'Why now?'

Stressed staff are less able to respond to, or deal with, challenging or potentially violent situations, which consequentially occur more frequently and seriously. Organisational, funding and educational changes within the National Health Service (NHS) clearly have impacted upon the relationship between patients and staff, as well as that of the organisation and its staff. There has been a major drive to meet politically determined targets and implement policies for which there is little evidence of support from nurses. Some of these have undoubtedly increased stress levels and the difficulties in their relationship, as an occupational group, with their management. Open discussion of problems or any apparent form of dissent has been increasingly suppressed since the early 1990s, often by forms of autocratic and authoritarian management, for example, 'gagging clauses'. This prevents problems being resolved and staff respond by feeling increasingly frustrated, resentful and angry, commonly expressed as stress, which, unfortunately, completes a cycle of nurses being less able to respond to challenging behaviours and situations with patients (Hart, 2004).

Risk assessment

When assessing challenging behaviours, it is important to know why it has presented as a problem at this time, as this can help identify the actual problem that needs to be addressed (Table 4.2).

It is vital to identify what risks, actual and potential, result from the behaviour. A specific risk assessment is required, associated with the behaviour, but should incorporate a wider perspective, for example, the behaviour might be occurring on the ward but is the patient likely to leave and, if so, will the behaviour and risks decrease or increase? These considerations will influence the team's response.

An organisational response to challenging behaviours

The concept of 'zero tolerance' raises a number of practical problems. First, it is difficult to enforce if a patient requires treatment and care. Second, the police are reluctant to intervene in a hospital, particularly if there is any suspicion that the patient may have mental health problems and continuing problems with the wider criminal justice system. Zero tolerance also removes the need for nurses or other health workers to try to understand behaviours and the reactions of patients, while it assumes no responsibility lies with anyone other than the patient or individual. As outlined above, there are clear reasons why nurses are experiencing many incidences of challenging behaviour and worse. There is obviously a need for clear boundaries and an understanding

Table 4.2 Factors to consider when assessing challenging behaviours.

Factors to consider before assessment	Where will the assessment be carried out? Is it safe for those involved? If not, what steps need to be taken to ensure everyone's safety?
What has prompted the assessment at this time?	What recent event(s) precipitated or triggered this presentation or made you think assessment was necessary now? Does the person pose an immediate (i.e. within the next few minutes or hours) risk with specific plans to self-harm or aggression/violence towards you or others? Is there any suggestion, or does it appear likely, that the person may try to abscond?
What is the actual problem?	Is there a clear description of the behaviour and understanding of why it is a problem? For whom is it a problem? Is there a pattern to this behaviour? Is there an underlying cause, e.g. organic, drug and/or alcohol intoxication (or withdrawal), mental illness? Has anything worked in the past to reduce or stop the behaviour?
Past history	Does the person have a history of violence? Is there a history of self-harm?
Perceptions	Does the patient have any psychotic ideas (see Chapter 10)? What is the patient's perception of the problem? Does the person feel he has any control over the situation?
Cognition	Does the person have the capacity to consent, i.e. can the patient understand and retain information, and then make balanced judgements based on an evaluation of his options?
Risk	What are the risks? How immediate is the risk? What would be the likely impact of any actions if the person were to act upon his ideas?
Formulation	What is your understanding of the issues the patient has described? What is the level of risk? Is immediate action required? For example, action to make the situation safe, such as involving security staff, or contacting the police Is a referral to the mental health liaison team necessary and, if so, how urgent is it?

Table 4.3 Three stages in the clinical management process to minimise challenging behaviours.

Stage 1: Pro-active
Maintain an environment that is as calm and as peaceful as possible
Provide patients with information and materials to relieve boredom
Maintain good systems of open communications
Identify nurses and other clinicians/support staff as people rather as 'anonymous' staff
Offer flexibility within clear boundaries
Take an attentive approach, both in listening and in communicating
Prioritise time to get to know patients' individual needs
Have ongoing training and education programmes, particularly around mental health issues
Hold multi-disciplinary team reviews of all patients and routinely involve patients in decisions about their treatment and care
Provide clinical supervision
Develop and use problem-solving forums, e.g. shared governance councils

Stage 2: Intermediate
Provide regular training in risk assessment, de-escalation techniques and conflict transformation (see below)
Have access to specialist supervision around particular patients and/or situations (this is a service that most mental health liaison teams can provide) – see Chapter 6

Stage 3: Crisis
Have up-to-date and effective alarm systems
Have staff trained in safe procedures for managing violence and aggression
Ensure clinicians are aware of the rapid tranquilisation policy
Utilise the criminal justice system when appropriate

of what behaviour is acceptable, as well as measures to address wrong-doing. But a blanket approach to every situation, assuming they are all the same, negates the complexity of the health care situation and human relationships. It is also reacting after an incident has occurred, whereas a measured, pro-active approach that addresses patients' clinical needs and the organisational needs of health care staff is required to be effective (Table 4.3).

Providing staff support is paramount, as this will influence the quality of the care and communication that the person receives. If staff feel confident and able to achieve their goals and have some perspective on their work, with as little organisational conflict as possible, they will be better equipped to address internal conflicts and any conflicts that occur with patients.

Working with people who challenge us

Environmental, educational and organisational factors are only enablers – it is the nurse–patient relationship, finally, which is going to minimise the

Table 4.4 Key skills and approaches in providing care for the person displaying challenging behaviour.

Offer a consistent framework of care and treatment

Minimise splitting by keeping the same nurses working with the patient and using care plans they have agreed with him or, if he would not agree, that he is aware of

Find out reasons for non-adherence and address these with the patient

Set clear limits, but emphasise what is available if the person stays within them

Give positive rewards for non-challenging behaviour, but do not react to challenging behaviour unless necessary and then do so consistently

Look at previous negative experiences and work with the patient to see if he can identify differences from his current treatment and care

Take an unbiased look at the person's requirements and criticisms

Acknowledge the feelings of the patient

Demonstrate empathy (see Chapter 1)

Employ anxiety management techniques (as anxiety will underlie most challenging behaviours)

Teach new behaviours, such as assertiveness and interpersonal effectiveness

Provide more information, if that is what the patient is seeking and there is information to give

Make use of clinical supervision

---

problems and disruption attributed to challenging behaviour. If nurses are given the opportunity, and are able to employ the range of skills and attributes integral to this core element of their role, particularly engaging the patient in a meaningful negotiation about the care and treatment he is to receive, then everything will be easier. This is not to suggest there will never be problems, but such behaviour is often a symptom of the relationship that forms when caring for people.

Many of these skills are identified and referred to in Chapter 1. However, those listed below are more specific to the issues of caring for a patient while he is displaying a challenging behaviour (Table 4.4). Conflict resolution has been recognised as a key skill in this area, with a range of techniques identified. These include:

- Denial of the conflict or withdrawal from it
- Suppression or 'smoothing over'
- The use of power or dominance
- Compromise or negotiation
- Integration or collaboration.

This latter approach is often the most successful, with the emphasis on trying to solve the problem at hand, rather than in defending particular positions or factions. The expectation of modifying original views is encouraged. The others all run the risk of apparently resolving the conflict but leaving one or both parties dissatisfied, which can obviously be grounds for further conflict, even if this is unacknowledged.

Conflict transformation is concerned primarily with changing the attitudes and perceptions of the parties to one another. It seeks to work at a much deeper level of the human psyche than previous models of conflict resolution, working on the assumption that merely co-operating to generate 'win-win solutions' to conflict does not change underlying attitudes, which may easily resurface and fuel other conflicts (Salla, 2000).

Embedded negative images are a serious obstacle to conflict management, routinisation, reduction, or resolution. Once formed, these images tend to become deeply rooted and resistant to change, even when the object of challenging behaviour attempts to signal a change in intent. The images themselves then perpetuate and intensify the conflict.

In a clinical situation, it might mean that a nurse approaches a patient and offers a particular intervention which might be assumed to be helpful and for which the nurse might expect the patient to be receptive. However, for the patient, it might act as a reminder of an earlier situation in which he was deeply unhappy or felt let down, perhaps by another carer. This can lead to a rejection of the nurse's offer and set the stage for difficulties in the relationship. The conflict, therefore, has to be taken as an opportunity to transform the patient's perceptions and feelings to prevent future conflicts with other nurses or health care professionals. It involves taking a more radical approach to change the underlying emotions and perceptions that influence the behaviour. Systematic efforts can be made to get those involved to acknowledge and identify each other's feelings, needs and perceptions, and to seek to improve these. Identifying these elements in an open way can often be a major step forward in itself. It then offers the opportunity for a conflict situation to be satisfactorily dealt with. The stage is then set for dealing with any legitimate issues and concerns the patient or, indeed, the nurse may have. In this context empathy is so important, enabling the nurse to demonstrate an understanding of the patient's position, what it is like for him and what the process of change might entail. This is obviously more complex and time consuming than some other forms of conflict resolution. In some clinical areas it is not going to be possible to go through such a transformative process simply because the patient may not be there long enough. In this respect, nurses should try to develop a range of conflict resolution and transformation skills and an awareness of their appropriateness to a particular situation.

Conclusions

The source of much of the conflict or challenging behaviours nurses face lies in the context of the nurse–patient relationship. However, organisational and educational issues, and the huge stress of the work of caring, all contribute to how well the nurse responds. The 'difficult' patient is, in most cases, an embodiment of wider institutional problems of our creation, whether or not the individual is a 'willing participant'. Moreover, it is a matter of people developing challenging behaviours as a response to a frightening or frustrating situation they perceive as being beyond their control. They then use an array of psychological and behavioural mechanisms to attempt to wrest control in a highly maladaptive manner that exacerbates the situation. The role of the nurse is vital, therefore, not just to the needs of the patient but the effective working of the wider organisation. Paradoxically, it is the effective role of the hospital in supporting the nurse in this aspect of her work that makes it manageable and achievable, and calls for a fundamental re-evaluation of the involvement of nurses in key decision-making.

References

Brandon, D. (1990) *Zen in the Art of Helping*. London: Penguin.

Breeze, J.A. & Repper, J. (1998) Struggling for control: the care experiences of 'difficult' patients in mental health services. *Journal of Advanced Nursing*, 28 (6): 1301–1311.

Casement, P. (1986) *On Learning from the Patient*. London: Routledge.

Cobbs, P.M. (1975) The victim's perspective. In: J. Howard & A. Strauss (eds) *Humanising Health Care*. Berkeley: University of California Press.

Coulson, J. & Carr, C.T. (1976) *Oxford Illustrated Dictionary*. Oxford: Oxford University Press.

Dexter, G. & Walsh, M. (1995) *Psychiatric Nursing Skills: a patient centred approach*. London: Chapman and Hall.

Gatward, N. (1997) Managing the 'manipulative' patient – a different perspective. *Nursing Standard*, 13 (22): 36–38.

Geisler, L. (1991) *Doctor and Patient – a partnership through dialogue*. Frankfurt: Pharma Verlag.

Gournay, K. (2002) *The Recognition, Prevention and Therapeutic Management of Violence*. London: NMC.

Hantikainen, V. (2001) Nursing staff perceptions of the behaviour of older nursing home residents and decision making on restraint use: a qualitative and interpretative study. *Journal of Clinical Nursing*, 10 (2): 246–256.

Hart, C. (2004) *Nurses and Politics: the impact of power and practice*. Basingstoke: Palgrave Macmillan.

Linehan, M.M. (1993) *Skills Training for Treating Borderline Personality Disorder*. New York: Guildford Press.

Obholzer, A. & Roberts, V.R. (1994) The troublesome individual and the troubled institution. In: A. Obholzer & V.R. Roberts (eds) *The Unconscious at Work: individual and organisational stress in the human services*, pp. 129–138. London: Routledge.

Perlin, C.K. (2001) Social responses and personality disorders. In: G.W. Stuart & M.T. Laraia (eds) *Principles and Practice of Psychiatric Nursing*. St Louis: Mosby.

Ridley, M. (1993) *The Red Queen: sex and the evolution of nature*. London: Macmillan.

Ritvo, M.M. (1963) Who are 'good' and 'bad' patients? *Modern Hospital*, 100 (6): 79–81.

Salla, M.E. (2000) Conflict resolution, genetics and alchemy – the evolution of conflict transmutation. *The Online Journal of Peace and Conflict Resolution*, Issue 3.3, June 2000. www.trinstitute.org

Slevin, O. (2003) A nursing perspective on older people: the problem of ageism. In: L. Basford & O. Slevin (eds) *Theory and Practice of Nursing*. Bath: Nelson Thornes.

Smith, P. (1992) *The Emotional Labour of Nursing*. Basingstoke: Macmillan.

Stuart, G.W. (2001) Anxiety responses and anxiety disorders. In: G.W. Stuart & M.T. Laraia (eds) *Principles and Practice of Psychiatric Nursing*. St Louis: Mosby.

Sundeen, S.J., Stuart, G.W. & Rankin, E.A.D. (1998) *Nurse–Client Interaction: implementing the nursing process*. St Louis: Mosby.

Chapter 5
Breaking Bad News

Chapter aims

> ### This chapter will:
>
> - define what is meant by 'bad news' and why it may be interpreted as such
> - describe the factors that contribute to an individual's understanding and interpretation of bad news
> - discuss the processes involved in providing information and assessing individual understanding in relation to bad news
> - discuss the various responses to bad news by patients and carers
> - discuss the professional and ethical issues involved in imparting bad news.

Introduction

The notion of breaking 'bad news' poses a number of challenges. First, and most importantly, how do we know that the news we are about to impart will be perceived by the patient as 'bad'? A patient may receive definite news – whether or not it is perceived by clinicians as 'bad' – as conferring a degree of certainty and be grateful for this, particularly if it confirms a long held suspicion or belief. Equally, information that the bearer may have thought of as being relatively unimportant could have had a severe impact on the patient and/or family members.

There is also the question of who should tell the patient the particular news. Is it best delivered by someone who knows him? Or should it be the person who has all the information available, to cover any question the patient and/or relatives may wish to ask? Should it be the consultant, as the person with overall responsibility for the patient's treatment, or is there a 'specialist' in such matters as breaking bad news? The breaking of bad news is most closely associated with having to tell a patient he has a terminal illness and faces death. As such, much of the literature comes from the areas of critical care and palliative care. However, it is work which nurses in all clinical areas should be equipped for, as there are undoubtedly many occasions when they will be called upon to break bad news. This chapter will seek to answer these questions, as well as define best practice in this difficult area.

What is bad news?

In a health care setting, typically accepted cases of bad news would be informing someone of a significant loss. An example might be telling someone they have sustained a life-changing injury or contracted a debilitating disease, terminal illness or that their illness is worse in some way than previously thought. Buckman (1984) defined bad news as new information that drastically and negatively alters the patient's view of his future. Ptacek and Eberhardt (1996) expanded on this, stating that bad news results in cognitive, behavioural or emotional deficits in the recipient which lasts beyond the period when they received the news itself. More simply, Farrell (1999) defined bad news as 'the news of life-threatening illness, disability or impending or actual death'.

It can be said to depend on the patient's existing view of his health, as well as what he knows or thinks about his future. However, information is integrated into what are obviously individualised belief systems. A nurse may know that a particular condition or development in a patient's treatment is not highly significant but, for the patient, this may have a very specific, distressing meaning. For instance, a relatively minor illness may have presaged something far more serious in someone the patient was close to. The patient may believe that something the nurse thinks is relatively minor can actually be life threatening.

Clearly, it is not possible to work with every patient on the premise that every piece of information may be construed as bad news. As will be explored further, the most effective way around this is, wherever possible, to spend time getting to know the patient at an early stage in his admission, particularly finding out what he knows about his illness or why he has been admitted to hospital. Eliciting details of any past medical history can include questions about any particular fears or experiences with doctors or nurses that might give a hint to potential problem areas. Looking at the family history and illnesses within the family may also reveal concerns about particular fears, however irrational these might appear.

As the patient's treatment and care progress, it may also emerge that they have particular anxieties about the consequences of an illness or condition. So it may be that telling someone they are going to have an operation is of enormous consequence and would most definitely qualify as bad news for them. Equally, a clinical development that would require prolonged hospitalisation, incapacity or a particular type of treatment could all, easily, fall into this category. Indeed, being told of a serious health condition or injury can constitute, of itself, bad news, given that ill health is known to bring social and economic marginalisation (Buckman, 1992).

The manner in which bad news is presented will affect the way in which the patient develops an understanding of their condition and their adjustment to it (Stewart *et al.*, 1999) and only emphasises the benefits of developing good techniques for doing so.

Issues of grief and loss

Elizabeth Kubler-Ross (1969) wrote about a lack of knowledge about and, consequently, difficulty in caring for the dying, famously describing what were interpreted as five stages of death: denial, anger, bargaining, depression and acceptance, although these were originally identified, far more appropriately, as the five stages of receiving catastrophic news. Kubler-Ross' theories were engulfed in controversy by the end of the century, with thanatologists such as Michelle Chaban (2004) and journalists such as Robertson (1999) heavily criticising both her theories and their effectiveness, while also claiming that her work was poorly researched and took generously, but uncredited, from the efforts of others, particularly a Chicago chaplain called Carl Nighswonger (Robertson, 1999).

Despite the criticisms, there is no doubt that Kubler-Ross' work opened up the debate about how to deal with the breaking of bad news and the issue of death. In the 1950s and 1960s, 88% of physicians indicated a preference for not telling patients about a diagnosis of cancer (Oken, 1961), while there were even published methods for deceit (Buckman, 1984). There has, however, been a recognition that the grief process is more complex, unique to the individual and that it can do more harm than good to try to 'shoehorn' the patient into a structured – and limited – series of responses (see Box 5.1).

Box 5.1 Emotions and reactions noted to be missing from the five stage model.

- Fear
- Guilt
- Anxiety
- 'Gallows' humour
- Shock
- Sadness
- Negotiating
- Hope
- Despair

There have been a number of attempts at defining grief. One simple equation identified is: change = loss = grief (Buckman, 1984).[1] Thus a change of circumstances of almost any kind leads to a feeling of loss, which, in turn, produces a grief reaction. Kastenbaum (1998) offers that bereavement is an objective fact, but it has to be remembered that if we are looking at cases where the patient is the recipient of bad news, that will not always be the case. The grief reaction is an internal, subjective response to the event, which is why it will vary from individual to individual – even close siblings will experience the loss of a parent differently – in terms of intensity, duration and factors that will assist in its resolution. Mourning can be seen as a signal of distress in the light of this painful response to loss or bereavement (Kastenbaum, 1998). However, it needs to be remembered that grief is a natural reaction and one that should not be unnecessarily pathologised. Stuart and Sundeen (1983) note that 'uncomplicated grief runs a consistent course that is modified by the abruptness of the loss, one's preparation for the event, and the significance of the lost object'. The delayed reaction or the distorted reaction imply something pathological or maladaptive.

Buckman (1992) has noted that the response is likely to be one of a simultaneous range of emotions rather than a series but has also identified a three stage model of the process of dying (Table 5.1).

Even such terms as 'not distressed' and 'normal' have to be qualified in this context, and the nurses who know the patient relatively well by the time he approaches death, and are experienced in caring for terminally ill patients, may well be equipped to help the patient with emotional responses that are often difficult, and behavioural reactions and difficulties making decisions

Table 5.1 The three stage model of the process of dying.

Stage	Process
Initial stage	'Facing the threat', characterised by a mixture of emotions, a time when the patient may be quite labile in mood and behaviour
Chronic stage	'Being ill', as the initial reaction resolves and the emotional intensity diminishes. Depressive symptoms become a possibility
Final stage	'Acceptance', defined by the patient's acceptance of death but not an essential state, providing the patient is not distressed, is communicating normally and making decisions normally

[1] This is, of course, a peculiarly Western perspective. Many Eastern religions and philosophies, especially Buddhism and Hinduism, highlight the impermanence of the human condition and place great emphasis on the lifelong preparation for death. See, for example, *The Tibetan Book of Living and Dying* (Rinpoche, 1992). Nonetheless, there is evidence that despite prevailing cultural and religious beliefs, the fear of death is pervasive and universal (Becker, 1973).

that would have been far easier with the person before the present situation developed. Acceptance may be achieved by the patient but clinicians should beware of an almost persecutory approach to helping the patient towards this goal when, for him, it is always likely to be unattainable, particularly if those involved have a pre-conceived notion of what that might be.

How people 'hear' what is said and 'understand' – the difference between being told something and understanding

In a busy hospital environment, a patient can often feel overwhelmed and struggle to keep pace with what is going on. Information can be relayed from clinicians to both the patient and relatives or carers and, once given, assumed to have been understood. However, only 30% of information is usually retained under normal circumstances (Kessels, 2003) and there is evidence that people often miss out on much of what has been said once an initial diagnosis is offered, 'presumably because they are in shock and focusing on the implications of what they have heard' (Ptacek & Ellison, 2000). Eden *et al.* (1994) found that patients' relatives did not always think they had been given information, even when the clinicians involved had recorded it for them, and concluded that relatives' emotional state can affect their ability to comprehend and retain the information provided for them.

Breaking bad news cannot be seen as a 'one off' intervention; there is a need, not just in the initial discussion, to make use of techniques such as reiteration, to return to the subject, make recordings for the patient and leave information with him that he can reflect upon. In checking that the person has an understanding, the nurse can use the 'capacity test', which is one framework that can be used for assessing the ability of the person to retain and process the information provided (see Chapter 3) (Department of Health, 2001):

- Does the patient understand what he has been told?
- Can he retain the information?
- Can he weigh up his options on the basis of the information given?
- Can he make a clear decision, with an understanding of the implications of that decision?

Even if he has been able to do all of that, it does not automatically mean that the person has 'understood' the information. Understanding has to take account of the impact of the information and is person-specific, for example, some people may never 'understand' the information given to them in the sense that they can recall it precisely and demonstrate that they know how it will affect them and their loved ones. However, a patient may nonetheless reach a level of understanding that means something personal to him and, in such cases, the nurse can document that the patient has taken in and made his own sense of the information given to him. Even then, as we shall discuss later, it is important to return to the issues that have been discussed, not just to see if the patient has retained his understanding but to continue the dialogue and provide the kind of emotional and psychological care required.

Preparing to provide information

Initially, even before thinking about what information to give the patient, there has to be clarity about why the information should be given. As has been stated, it was not so long ago that physicians (who are still the main bearers of bad news) routinely withheld bad news, believing it would be damaging for the patient (Oken, 1961). However, as the model has shifted from one of paternalism to patient autonomy, the issue arises of the patient who specifically does not wish to be told bad news. Inherent within the whole process, of course, is the tricky position of the clinician having to raise the subject in the first place, which inevitably is going to arouse concerns for the patient. Nonetheless, it is important to give the patient the opportunity to make his views about what information he might wish to receive, how and with who in attendance, at the earliest point possible in his treatment.

The clarity of what is said, the way in which it is said and the environment in which the discussion takes place will all have a significant impact on relationships between the clinical team, the patient and his carers (Farrell, 1999). In deciding what to say, there is also a need to place this in the context of what the patient already knows. This requires both knowing the patient and having access to good documentation from fellow clinicians. In the absence of either of these, it is as good to simply ask the patient what he knows, although care is needed as there is some evidence that patients pick up on unintentional cues and patterns of behaviour from health professionals and make assumptions on these cues (Arber & Gallagher, 2003). There will also be a different response to the question, 'What have you been told about your condition?' to 'What do you think about your condition?' or 'What do you think will happen with your illness?' all of which seek to explore the patient's ideas and feelings or interpretation about their condition, which may be very different from the 'reality' as it is understood by the clinicians.

It may be that the patient will ask a surprise question about his condition and the nurse may feel unready to respond. Rather than bluffing one's way through such a situation, giving a little – or incorrect – information, or suggesting that the patient needs to talk to a doctor, it is best to ask if the patient wants to speak to you particularly and, if so, acknowledge the importance of the conversation and arrange to return to discuss it in detail at the earliest opportunity. Patients may ask a clinician to whom they feel particularly close or in whom they have confidence. They may choose a student nurse or a health care assistant, perhaps because they may find them easier to talk to or because they assume they don't know that much about the detail of their condition and, therefore, wouldn't have access to unwelcome news (Arber & Gallagher, 2003).

There can now be very little to support arguments for a paternalistic decision not to tell patients about their condition and the ethical issues that arise out of such a decision, although Clark (2001) argues, as a doctor, that it is still better to withhold information from the older person facing death because it is too upsetting. It is far more complex, however, when thinking about what may be told to relatives and carers if the patient wants information withheld or only to be passed on to select individuals, particularly if the team think that the relatives need an opportunity to address end of life issues with the patient. There is, again, no formulaic response to this but it is one that can be discussed with the patient, whose preference must be recognised and, ultimately, confidentiality maintained (Nursing and Midwifery Council, 2004) if the matter cannot be resolved. A number of frameworks and protocols for breaking bad news have been identified (Box 5.2) (Buckman, 1992; Girgis & Sanson-Fisher, 1995; Kaye, 1996).

There is no one member of the clinical team who should do the telling. Historically, it was usually doctors who would break the bad news (Dunniece

---

Box 5.2 A framework for breaking bad news.

Gathering information. Finding out what the patient knows, what he wants to know and what the facts are that need to be relayed

Discussion with team. Deciding who is most appropriate to impart the news, when and where the discussion should take place and who else might be present

Preparing the physical environment. Ensuring the discussion can take place in a quiet, private environment where there will not be any interruptions, as well as allowing enough time to have a genuine two way discussion, with the patient having the opportunity to ask questions

Leading gently into the conversation. An opening statement such as, 'I have something serious to discuss with you regarding your illness/the results of the latest test results . . .' signals that there is bad news on the way but allows the patient to begin preparing himself

Using higher level communication skills. Open questions, such as 'How do you feel about hearing what I've said?' are going to be more helpful in eliciting the patient's feelings. However, a variety of questioning techniques will be required, helping the clinician to clarify, reiterate information already given, move the discussion forward or get it back on track if the patient is struggling, yet not leave him feeling that he has not been heard or that his views have been dismissed or trivialised. Other factors such as making eye contact and using a soft, quiet tone of voice can help maintain the patient's confidence (Farrell, 1999). Visual aids can be considered for people with a learning disability and interpreters when anyone for whom English is their second language or anyone who has a hearing disability has to be considered

Listening for cues to the patient's emotional reaction. The reaction of the patient is going to be unique to the individual. It is important to begin the process of asking questions and noting verbal and non-verbal cues as to how he feels even while the news is being given. It may be, for example, that the patient feels he needs to stop the discussion at some point and resume it at a later stage

Engaging and aligning. Once the news has been given, engaging with the patient's agenda, what he wants and why, how he wants to be cared for and treated, are known as aligning oneself with the patient (Maynard, 1989)

Normalising. Communicate to the patient and carers that the emotions and behaviours associated with grief are a normal process in the reaction to bad news and that, with time and the opportunity to work through the emotions and issues that arise, there will be a more positive change, although there may be a need to assist in helping the patient distinguish between acceptable behaviours (as opposed to acceptable emotional responses) and adaptive, rather than maladaptive, responses (Buckman, 1992)

Summarising. Towards the end of the discussion, it is useful to go over the key points again, and check whether or not the person wants further information, or to discuss anything in more detail

Begin the process of developing a plan. This is not something that can necessarily be developed there and then. The patient needs to be involved in this, but may need time to reflect upon what he has been told, possibly confer with relatives and come back and talk to the clinical team further. However, emphasising that a plan will be developed and then ensuring that one is developed will be important in helping the patient hold on to some degree of hope and confidence in the team

Arrange a follow up session. This will not only allow the facilitation of a plan but give the patient an opportunity to return to any questions that arose after the initial discussion and to his subsequent feelings

Leave further information. This might be a written record of the key points of the discussion – or even a tape. Leaflets from self-help or voluntary groups might be made available, as well as website addresses and anything else that might help the patient

& Slevin, 2000), although nurses might have been involved by sitting in on the discussions and were often left to 'pick up the pieces' afterwards (Walker *et al.*, 1996; Hart, 2004). For, although patients are more frequently told the truth about their condition, it is not always done very well, perhaps because there is no definitive evidence about best practice (Salander, 2002). As has been noted, this is highly intensive emotional labour and is not one that nurses or doctors are educated in, either in their pre or post graduate training. Contemporary thinking is that, wherever possible, the best person to do this is the clinician who has a good relationship with the patient (Farrell,

1999), although that needs to be qualified by noting that the clinician should have been trained in breaking bad news and have access to a support network within the clinical setting in which she works.

There are, of course, going to be occasions when the situations in which the clinician finds herself are very different, for instance, when someone dies in the emergency department (ED) and the family have to be told or, even more exceptionally, disasters or when people are involved in 'mass' situations, with media attention. Or it may be a case of a patient arriving in the department with a very serious condition or having had a bad accident. In such cases, it is highly unlikely that the nurse will know much about the patient and/ or family at all, which obviously negates the gathering of information and building on an existing relationship. Nonetheless, many of the principles outlined above will still apply, particularly about the discussion and how that is managed and ended, with the offer of follow up if the person feels the need for it, either to be conducted by you and the ED team or to be provided elsewhere, for example, by the person's general practitioner. Table 5.2 provides a summary of the principles of imparting bad news.

Table 5.2 A summary of 'dos and don'ts' when breaking bad news.

Do	Don't
Be guided by what the patient has said he wants to know about the disease process, treatment and prognosis	Impart bad news simply because you are aware of it
Think through and prepare carefully what it is you want to communicate, thinking about body language and non-verbal cues as much as what you'll say	Rush into telling the patient because the opportunity seems to present itself or you are asked an awkward question
Find out what the patient already knows about his condition and his perception of what that means for him	Assume you know what the patient knows
Have the available information about the patient's condition and possible options	Begin the discussion without having adequately prepared
Gather together any relatives/carers the patient would like present	Begin without knowing who people in the room are, whether the patient wants them to know or if there is someone he would want present but is not
Prepare the physical environment in which the discussion will take place	Allow interruptions or bleeps to go off
Use simple language with as little jargon as possible	Use jargon
Actively listen	

Table 5.2 (*Cont'd*)

Do	Don't
Find out the patient's agenda and align yourself, without giving up your agenda and the need to provide information	Trivialise the news or the patient's experience, e.g. 'Everything will be all right' or 'I'm sure you'll cope very well'
Lead up to the key news you want to impart	Become defensive or critical of others involved in the patient's treatment and care
Clarify the patient's understanding of what has been said	Reassure, e.g. telling the patient 'things will be all right', or 'not to worry'
Use reiteration	Make assumptions
Use – and tolerate – short silences	Allow insufficient time for the discussion
Explore the patient's feelings and reaction	Leave the patient without having checked what ongoing support they think they may need
Use open questions, always listening for cues from the patient	Use closed questions. They don't give the patient the option to talk freely
Use diagrams to illustrate difficult technical concepts or anatomical information	Assume the patient always understands what you're saying, particularly if the information is complex
Leave written information for the patient and carers to look at	Assume the patient has absorbed all the information in one session
Tell him about other sources of information, e.g. the internet, self-help organisations and leaflets	See above
Document, in detail, what has been discussed and report back to the rest of the multi-disciplinary team	Underestimate the importance of clear communication on such an important piece of work
Follow up the initial discussion	See above

Impact on practitioners

Breaking bad news is not simply another conversation with a patient. It is sharing with him something utterly unique and, on each occasion, is the beginning of a particular journey for that patient which the nurse will find herself sharing, at least a small part of. It involves the nurse confronting her own powerful emotions, which typically might include:

- guilt about the 'failure' of the treatment and the science underpinning it
- the fear of being blamed by the patient and/or carers

- not knowing enough to answer all of the patient's questions
- having insufficient skills and knowledge to carry out the task
- not being able to 'manage' emotions
- the fear of upsetting the patient or causing him further emotional pain.

There are, of course, our own fear of death, our own experiences of being given bad news about relatives and the impact on us of both the news itself and the way in which it was delivered. Although rarely acknowledged in the clinical arena, there is also the inevitable distress of having to talk to someone about the end of their life or significant and adverse changes to it. Smith (1992) has noted that this kind of emotional labour – essentially caring – does not come naturally and nurses have to work on themselves emotionally to give the impression of caring, irrespective of how they personally feel about themselves, individual patients, their circumstances and condition. They can also be taught to manage their feelings more effectively, although the work with the seriously ill and dying is something nurses also learn from watching more experienced colleagues, just as patients and relatives watch nurses to learn the same thing (Hart, 2004). It is incumbent upon the organisation as a whole, and the teams in which nurses work in particular, that they are supported in these endeavours, initially by specialist training and then by the type of support that clinical supervision can offer, in which the nurse can talk about her own experience of breaking bad news, build upon her experience but also resolve some of the emotional issues arising.

Conclusions

Breaking bad news is never easy. It is made more difficult by the unique, very human relationship that is involved between the patient, the subject of the 'bad news' and the clinician imparting it. It is a difficult task to give bad news and provide for the psychological, spiritual and emotional needs of the patient in the aftermath, as well as providing physical care, and the needs of nurses and other clinicians doing such work must be recognised by the clinical team as well as the institution. This is emotional labour at its most demanding and is one of the things that sets nursing apart from almost any other work (Hart, 2004).

There also has to be a recognition that, for all the preparation and education that might be given in this area, breaking bad news is rarely a neat and tidy experience and nor is death. The notion that everything will be done 'properly', it will be 'successful' and the patient will respond in some kind of synchronised order and find true acceptance and peace in the wake of the news, or before death, speaks more about an unrealistic but still prevalent model of medical and scientific control and the anxieties of the clinician.

As with so much else in nursing, any success that will be obtained is more in the process of breaking bad news. Saunders and Baines (1983) noted that it is as much the attempt to understand a patient and family's situation as any success in doing so which is interpreted as demonstrating the nurse's commitment to care, and the best predictor of patient satisfaction is the patient's perception that he is valued and cared about (Ptacek & Ellison, 2000).

The work that nurses do with patients in times of crisis, as they face the challenges of chronic or terminal illness and approach death, when it is done well, not only provides the patient with a realistic and genuine sense of hope and creates a sense of confidence in the clinical team, it is at the very heart of what nursing is about.

References

Arber, A. & Gallagher, A. (2003) Breaking bad news revisited: the push for negotiated disclosure and changing practice implications. *International Journal of Palliative Nursing*, 9 (4): 166–173.

Becker, E. (1973) *The Denial of Death*. New York: Free Press.

Buckman, R. (1984) *I Don't Know What to Say – how to help and support someone who is dying*. London: Papermac.

Buckman, R. (1992) *How To Break Bad News: a guide for health-care professionals*. London: Papermac.

Chaban, M. (2004) *The Life and Work of Dr Elisabeth Kubler-Ross and its Impact on the Death Awareness Movement*. New York: Edwin Mellen Press.

Clark, A.N.G. (2001) To tell or not to tell. *British Medical Journal*, 323: 489.

Department of Health (2001) *Reference Guide to Consent for Examination or Treatment*. London: DoH.

Dunniece, U. & Slevin, E. (2000) Nurses' experience of being present with a patient receiving a diagnosis of cancer. *Journal of Advanced Nursing*, 32 (3): 611–618.

Eden, O.B., Black, I. & MacKinley, G.A. (1994) Communication with parents of children with cancer. *Palliative Medicine*, 8: 105–114.

Farrell, M. (1999) The challenge of breaking bad news. *Intensive and Critical Care Nursing*, 15: 101–110.

Girgis, A. & Sanson-Fisher, R.W. (1995) Breaking Bad News: consensus guidelines for medical practitioners. *Journal of Clinical Oncology*, 13: 2449–2456.

Hart, C. (2004) *Nurses and Politics: the impact of power and practice*. Basingstoke: Palgrave Macmillan.

Kastenbaum, R.J. (1998) *Death, Society and Human Experience*, 6th edn., New York: Allyn & Bacon.

Kaye, P. (1996) *Breaking Bad News: a ten step approach*. Northampton: EPL Publications.

Kessels, R.P.C. (2003) Patient's memory for medical information. *Journal of the Royal Society of Medicine*, 96: 219–222.

Kubler-Ross, E. (1969) *On Death and Dying*. London: Macmillan.

Maynard, D. (1989) Notes on the delivery and reception of diagnostic news regarding mental disabilities. In: D.T. Helm, T. Anderson & J.A. Meehan (eds) *Directions in the Study of Social Disorder*. New York: Irvington.

Nursing and Midwifery Council (2004) *The NMC Code of Professional Conduct: standards for conduct, performance and ethics*. London: NMC.

Oken, D. (1961) What to tell cancer patients: a study of medical attitudes. *Journal of the American Medical Association*, 175: 1120–1128.

Ptacek, J.T. & Eberhardt, T.L. (1996) Breaking bad news: a review of the literature. *Journal of the American Medical Association*, 276: 496–502.

Ptacek, J.T. & Ellison, N. (2000) Health care providers' perspectives on breaking bad news to patients. *Critical Care Nursing Quarterly*, 23 (2): 51–59.

Rinpoche, S. (1992) *The Tibetan Book of Living and Dying*. London: Rider.

Robertson, H. (1999) Dead wrong. *Elm Street Magazine* (available at www.bereavement.org).

Salander, P. (2002) Bad news from the patient's perspective: an analysis of the written narratives of newly diagnosed cancer patients. *Social Science and Medicine*, 55 (5): 721–732.

Saunders, C. & Baines, M. (1983) *Living with Dying: the management of terminal illness*. Oxford: Oxford University Press.

Smith, P. (1992) *The Emotional Labour of Nursing*. Basingstoke: Macmillan.

Stewart, M., Brown, J.B. & Boon, H. (1999) Evidence on patient–doctor communication. *Cancer Prevention and Control*, 3 (1): 25–30.

Stuart, G.W. & Sundeen, S.J. (1983) *Principle and Practice of Psychiatric Nursing*. St Louis: Mosby.

Walker, G., Bradburn, J. & Maher, J. (1996) *Breaking Bad News*. London: King's Fund Publishing.

Chapter 6
The Role of the Mental Health Liaison Team

Chapter aims

> **This chapter will:**
>
> - describe the development of mental health liaison as a discrete speciality within the general hospital
> - identify the role and functions of the mental health liaison team
> - identify the contribution of the mental health liaison team to the provision of holistic health care within the general hospital
> - describe the role of general hospital staff in making a referral to the mental health liaison team.

Introduction

The development of mental health liaison services has occurred alongside the expansion of the mental health nurse's role into the general hospital. Since the early 1990s there has been a significant increase in the number of mental health liaison nurses (MHLNs) working within the general hospital. Liaison work is a generic term that can be applied to a wide variety of different settings, including liaison with primary care, police, non-statutory organisations such as drug and alcohol services, as well as between various hospital-based teams. For the purposes of this chapter, we define liaison as the practice of liaison and consultation that takes place between clinicians within the acute general hospital and staff of secondary care mental health services.

A comprehensive mental health liaison team (MHLT) should consist of a range of health and social care professionals, including doctors, nurses and psychologists. The role of the nurse is closely aligned to that of the doctor, although the main focus of nursing within such a team is the provision of mental health nursing assessment and intervention within the general hospital. Nurses undertaking a liaison role practise using the skills of consultation, liaison and collaborative working in order to provide a service that transcends traditional organisational and health service boundaries.

The development of mental health liaison practice

The term 'liaison nursing' as applied to the general hospital was first used in the United States during the 1960s (Jones, 1989), and it was here that the development of formal links between mental health and general hospitals became what is often known as 'liaison psychiatry'. The idea that mental health nurses can contribute to the care of patients while in the general hospital has also developed from the work of the nursing theorist Hildegard Peplau (1964). Peplau's model focuses on the development of the therapeutic relationship with the patient, something that is given priority within her theoretical framework, and is arguably of equal importance to all branches of nursing, whatever the speciality. Peplau's model emphasises holistic care and is of relevance to both mental health and non-mental health nurses, in that it provides a nursing framework that allows for the recognition, assessment and care of the person's psychological as well as physical state. Her work predates more recent service and professional developments in the UK that have seen an expansion in the number of nurses practising in the field of mental health liaison. In many instances the terms 'mental health liaison nursing' and 'mental health liaison' are used interchangeably.

Liaison psychiatry originated in the United States during the 1930s, and following World War II, services increased tenfold, with the most significant growth occurring during the 1960s and 1970s (Morriss & Mayou, 1996). In the UK informal liaison arrangements developed in some centres during the 1960s, but it was not until the late 1970s that psychiatrists became specifically interested in the mental health care of patients in the general hospital. This occurred at the same time as the development of community-based mental health services, brought about by the start of a huge programme of psychiatric hospital closures. Morriss and Mayou (1996), however, suggest that it was the decriminalisation of suicide in 1961 that provided the impetus for psychiatric teams to take more of an interest in the care of patients with physical illness. The then Ministry of Health advised that all individuals who attempted suicide should be assessed by a psychiatrist prior to being discharged from hospital; this is something that has been identified as good practice ever since, but remains an elusive goal for the majority of general hospitals.

On both continents, doctors (mostly psychiatrists) who had developed particular interests in certain illnesses, such as epilepsy and other neurological conditions, dominated early practice in the speciality. As with the medical profession, nursing in the United States led the way in the development of liaison practice. Mental health nursing posts within UK general hospitals were rare at this time and it was not until 1994 that there was formal recognition of the potentially valuable role that mental health nurses could play in the care of people with physical illness (Department of Health (DoH), 1994). Despite the length of time it took to recognise the potential role for mental health nurses in this setting, practitioners such as Jones (1989) and Tunmore (1990) described early examples of the role and its development in clinical practice across the UK.

The majority of early posts in mental health liaison were concerned with the assessment of patients following self-harm and attempted suicide, with nurses focusing on services to the Emergency Department (ED) (Tunmore, 1994). Although many practitioners now report working in a wide variety of clinical settings, the provision of self-harm assessments and the management of psychiatric emergencies via EDs continues to be the focus for many MHLNs (Loveridge & Carr, 1996; Roberts & Whitehead, 2002). Although the role of the mental health nurse within the general hospital can be seen as an autonomous and specialist role in its own right, the relatively slow development of posts is likely to have been influenced by the recommendation that liaison teams should only be developed secondary to the appointment of doctors (Royal College of Physicians/Royal College of Psychiatrists, 1995, 2003).

A problem for MHLNs and liaison practice generally has been the relative lack of co-ordinated service development or educational opportunities. Many services have grown up in a piecemeal fashion, often starting as single-practitioner services, with individuals employed to develop the role, function and service philosophy all at the same time. The lack of systematic development means that on the whole liaison services continue to lack the importance they deserve in respect of local health planning and commissioning (Lewis, 2004). The publication of the *National Service Framework for Mental Health* (NSF) in 1999 (DoH), helped to focus the attention of health planners on the provision of services for those patients with mental health needs who attend EDs in crisis, or as a result of self-harm. However, the NSF did not identify the other areas of psychiatric morbidity within the general hospital as requiring specific development, with the result that establishing comprehensive liaison arrangements in this area remains a challenge (Lewis, 2004).

The publication of guidelines relating to the management of specific conditions, such as self-harm and cancer (National Institute for Clinical Excellence (NICE), 2004a, b), has meant that welcome attention is being paid to the psychological needs of patients in the general hospital, although there continues to be a danger that self-harm is prioritised over other mental health problems. Increasingly NSFs are specifically addressing the psychological components of care (DoH, 2000, 2001). However, the ongoing challenge is to ensure that such standards are prioritised alongside the other milestones, as, despite the numerous recommendations cited in various reports and other publications, the provision of consistent and fully functioning mental health liaison services remains patchy across the UK.

Core elements of mental health liaison practice overlap with the recent development of crisis and home treatment services for individuals with

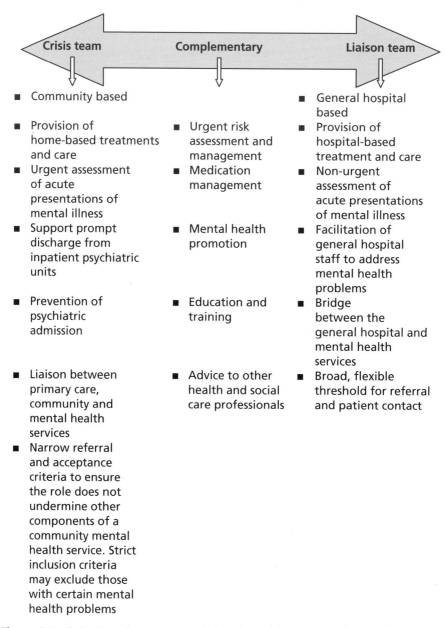

Figure 6.1 Distinctions between mental health crisis teams and mental health liaison teams.

mental health problems (Fig. 6.1). In some organisations, liaison roles and posts have been subsumed within models of mental health crisis provision, although as has been demonstrated in the preceding chapters, liaison practice within the general hospital has a unique and distinct focus. While there are occasions when individuals may present with acute and urgent mental health needs in the general hospital, the majority of an MHLT's practice should not be considered as urgent, i.e. as a mental health emergency. The risk inherent in merging MHLT roles with those of mental health crisis teams is that other legitimate mental health and psychological problems will be missed because they fall outside the scope of such services. It is only possible to address the range of psychological problems experienced by individuals with physical illness if there are specific MHLTs within each general hospital. The work of mental health crisis and home treatment teams should be considered as complementary to that of MHLTs, rather than as an alternative to them.

Staffing and skill mix within teams varies. Good practice is that each team should have a range of professionals, with core roles being those of medical and nursing staff. Clinical psychologists have been identified as having a potentially important role in such teams, in particular those who focus on the provision of specific psychological therapies such as cognitive behavioural therapy and motivational interviewing. Some teams may include social workers and occupational therapists, although there is a lack of clarity regarding the specific contribution of these professional groups within an MHLT. A few teams have consisted of an individual professional, such as a doctor or nurse, working in isolation (Callaghan *et al.*, 2002a).

Planning and commissioning of liaison services has generally been patchy and inconsistent, and there has been no strategic national agenda or guidance for health planners in this area. Although guidance for health purchasers has existed since 1995 (Royal College of Physicians/Royal College of Psychiatrists), the majority of commissioners have failed to translate this into the development of comprehensive and collaborative models of service. It is often tempting for senior health staff within a general hospital to approach individual mental health practitioners directly, with the aim of developing ad-hoc service level agreements to provide mental health input into a specific department or unit. Such service developments, while prompted by a genuine desire to improve the care patients receive, are often completely dependent upon the enthusiasm and good will of individual clinicians. Given the often arbitrary way in which such services develop, it could be argued that such an approach can never truly meet patient need in a systematic and holistic way. While the enthusiasm and commitment of the clinicians concerned cannot be questioned, such unplanned developments represent a clear failure of the health planning and commissioning processes. This position is supported by the increasing number of national reports and recommendations that advocate a collaborative approach to the provision of mental health care at the planning stages (NICE, 2004a).

The establishment of MHLTs within general hospitals has been shown to be a cost-effective way of addressing mental health problems in this setting. Evidence from the United States has shown that liaison teams can have a positive impact on factors such as overall length of hospital stay and patient and staff satisfaction (Levenson *et al.*, 1990). There are only limited data within the UK regarding the analysis of the cost-benefits of mental health liaison, although it is widely accepted that MHLTs have a huge potential to improve the utilisation and effectiveness of current health care resources within the general hospital (Lewis, 2004).

There has been limited investigation into the level of user satisfaction with mental health liaison services. Anecdotal evidence suggests that the majority of individuals value the service provided, although the nature of the contact and the impact of the environment are often issues that patients express dissatisfaction with. Attention to fundamental aspects of care, such as privacy, time to talk and improved written communication have been cited by patients as areas of liaison practice that need to be improved (Callaghan *et al.*, 2002b).

The role of the mental health liaison team

The prime function of the MHLT is the provision of a mental health assessment and intervention service to the general hospital. In order to undertake this effectively it is important that the team has clear goals and that each team member is able to develop effective relationships with colleagues. Certain characteristics will define an effective and dynamic MHLT (Table 6.1) and it is these that will ensure that the service is able to meet the needs of patients, carers and staff when practising in this setting.

As stated earlier, a major focus for many teams is the assessment and management of individuals attending or admitted following an episode of self-harm (Tunmore, 1997; Whitehead & Royles, 2002), although the MHLT has the potential to be involved in the care of a much wider group of patients. The potential for individuals to experience psychological distress following illness or injury is significant, and input from the MHLT has been shown to be particularly beneficial in specific clinical settings (Box 6.1).

The commonest reasons for referral to the MHLT will include:

- self-harm
- mood disorders, including depression and anxiety
- acute stress reactions
- disturbed, aggressive or 'bizarre' behaviour
- problems associated with excessive alcohol and illicit drug use
- confusional states and dementia.

Assessment is a core activity for all teams, with the majority of referrals being made with the expectation that a liaison practitioner will undertake direct client-centred work. The terms 'liaison' and 'consultation' are often used interchangeably, although they are in fact two distinct activities. Caplan (1970) was the first to describe in detail a theoretical model of liaison and consultation practice, covering four main domains of professional activity. His is a comprehensive model of consultation-liaison work, but it is likely that a relatively small number of MHLTs will be practising across all the domains identified. Within the UK, it is more common for teams to utilise specific

Table 6.1 Characteristics of an effective mental health liaison team.

Perequisites	Characterised by
Positive approach to mental health and the needs of people with mental health problems	A flexible and responsive service model, enabling prompt responses to requests for advice and assessment A low threshold for access to the service, with a straightforward referral mechanism Willingness to accept nurse-to-nurse referrals Ability to constructively challenge negative or patient-blaming attitudes concerning mental health

Detailed knowledge of mental health and psychiatric illness	Appropriately qualified and experienced personnel
	Competence in the following areas of practice:
	    Assessment
	    Risk assessment and management
	    Treatment – including psychopharmacology and medication management
	    Administration and documentation
	    Teaching and clinical supervision

Ability to deliver effective mental health care in non-mental health settings	Creative approach to mental health needs, e.g. arranging follow up and reassessment if necessary, ensuring individual patients receive a reassessment or review during their hospital stay; facilitating the development and implementation of effective care planning skills by non-mental health staff
Ability to identify areas where mental health needs go unrecognised and unmet	Participation in service planning and development with senior colleagues within the general hospital Preparation of reports and participation in meetings to inform the development and improvement of mental health care, e.g. *Essence of Care* benchmarking groups (DoH, 2003)

Box 6.1 Clinical settings where the provision of mental health liaison input is of particular benefit.

- Emergency departments
- Cardiology units
- Renal units
- Neurology units
- Cancer units
- Trauma units
- Transplant services
- Services for older people
- Sexual health units
- Perinatal units

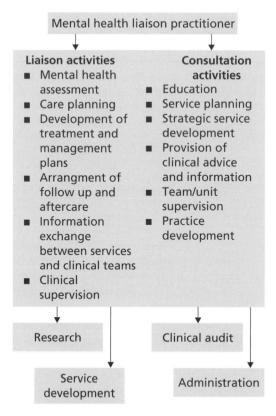

Figure 6.2 Overview of the liaison and consultation activities undertaken by mental health liaison teams.

elements of this model within their daily practice, as opposed to working fully within Caplan's framework.

Much of the work undertaken by MHLTs will involve face-to-face contact with individual patients, although many other activities, such as participation in care planning, providing advice and acting as a professional resource, can be broadly termed consultation activities. All mental health liaison practitioners should be skilled in both direct patient-focused work, or liaison, and indirect clinical activity, or consultation (Fig. 6.2).

In some instances it may be difficult for general hospital staff to develop a sense of clarity regarding the role of the MHLT, or to appreciate why they are making a referral in a particular situation. Sometimes a referral may be generated for no other reason than the practitioner has a sense of uncertainty regarding what is needed for the patient. An effective MHLT will operate with a low threshold for referral, encouraging early contact between teams if a mental health problem is suspected or detected. A valuable and essential aspect of the team's role is the provision of advice, information and guidance before individual problems become severe or entrenched. In order to assist in identifying the point at which an individual patient may need to be referred to the MHLT, the development of care guidance and care pathways provides an effective means of enabling staff to identify the severity of individual clinical problems (Harrison & Devey, 2003).

The process of referral

Referrals to the MHLT should be considered in the way that other referrals to specialist teams are undertaken. While the process of arranging a mental health assessment should not be overly complicated, it is important to remember that requesting specialist contact should never be undertaken lightly. Because of the nature of some mental health problems, individuals may present with symptoms that at first sight appear to be psychiatric in origin. Some of these problems, such as acutely disturbed behaviour, agitation and unco-operativeness, can lead practitioners to assume a mental illness, when in fact these types of behavioural symptoms are more frequently associated with an underlying organic or metabolic disturbance. Ensuring that all possible underlying causes of such behaviour have been excluded and treated before a referral to the MHLT is made is an important first step (Tables 6.2 and 6.3).

The referral process will vary from team to team, although all MHLTs should ensure that:

- They have an operational policy that clearly identifies the role and function of the team, alongside practical details such as how referrals to the team are received and allocated.
- There is a single point of entry to the team, thus avoiding arbitrary decisions by non-mental health staff regarding whether the person needs to be seen by a nurse, psychiatrist, psychologist, etc.
- There is a standard proforma that can be used to provide details of all referrals to the team.
- Clear standards exist regarding timescales (e.g. length of time between referral and assessment), provision of written information for professionals and patients, and the MHLT's role in relation to the provision of follow up while the patient remains in hospital.

All registered nursing staff should be aware of how to make a referral to an MHLT, ensuring that relevant information is included (Table 6.4). Before initiating a referral, it is important to ensure that this decision is one that has been reached after consultation and discussion within the clinical team. It is not good practice to make snap judgements, based on limited information or initial assessment, about the need for a mental health referral. The nurse has an important role to play in ensuring that all members of the clinical team are clear about the purpose and expectations of making such a referral. Good practice in this area consists of:

Table 6.2 Physical causes of common psychiatric symptoms.

Symptom	Possible physical cause
Depression	Cancer Infections Electrolye imbalance, e.g. low sodium level Endocrine disorders, e.g. hypothyroidism Neurological disorders, e.g. epilepsy, Parkinson's disease, dementia, stroke Addison's disease Autoimmune disease, e.g. systemic lupus erythematosus, rheumatoid arthritis
Anxiety	Endocrine disorders, e.g. hyperthyroidism Substance withdrawal, e.g. sudden cessation of benzodiazepines, sudden cessation of alcohol Hypoglycaemia Phaeochromocytoma Neurological disorders
Fatigue	Anaemia Sleep disorders, e.g. sleep apnoea Chronic infections Diabetes Endocrine disorders, e.g. hypothyroidism, Addison's disease, Cushing's syndrome Cancer Radiotherapy
Weakness	Autoimmune disease, e.g. myasthenia, rheumatoid arthritis Peripheral neuropathy Neurological disorders, e.g. Parkinson's disease
Headache	Migraine Brain tumours Temporal arteritis

- Ensuring that the reasons for a mental health referral are clear.
- Being familiar with the role of the MHLT in order that the nurse can answer the patient's questions or concerns about the need for a referral.
- Discussing the need for a mental health review with the patient and ensuring that, whenever possible, their views are sought, and their consent and co-operation are forthcoming. If the patient agrees, discussion with his or her family or significant other should take place.
- Ensuring that all the relevant history and background information is available and accessible before making the referral. For example, contacting the person's general practitioner (GP), obtaining collateral information from family members, community nursing teams and social care services (e.g. home support workers).

Table 6.3 Medications that can cause psychiatric side effects.

Side effect	Medication
Acute confusion, i.e. delirium	Central nervous system depressants, e.g. hypnotics, sedatives, antidepressants, antihistamines Antimuscarines, e.g. procyclidine Beta-blockers Digoxin Cimetidine
Psychotic symptoms	Appetite suppressants Beta-blockers Corticosteroids Levodopa Indometacin
Depression	Antihypertensives Oral contraceptives Antipsychotics Anticonvulsants Corticosteroids Levodopa
Elated mood	Antidepressants Corticosteroids Antimuscarines, e.g. benzhexol
Behavioural disturbance	Anaesthetic agents Benzodiazepines Antipsychotics Lithium toxicity

Table 6.4 Information that needs to be communicated to the MHLT as part of the referral process.

Patient information	Essential biographical details – name, address, date of birth, GP Hospital number Date of admission Note whether patient understands and is in agreement with the referral
Clinical information	Reason for admission to hospital Reason for referral – based on your assessment of the person's needs and discussions with the individual concerned, identify why you feel a mental health assessment is needed Brief overview of current treatments, in particular medication Degree of urgency

- Practising from a patient-centred perspective – ensuring that the reason for referral is motivated by a desire to improve the care available to the individual, as opposed to a reaction to systems failures within the hospital or team. Such systems failures can include issues such as a shortage of hospital beds, the assumed failure of nursing or residential homes to accept the transfer of the person back into their service once their physical care has been completed, breaches of waiting time 'targets', attaching labels, failure to interpret behaviour accurately, etc.
- Being clear of the expectations that you have of the MHLT before referral. For example, what do you hope will be the outcome of the assessment? This may include obtaining specialist advice regarding treatment or nursing care, participating in discharge planning by arranging mental health follow up or identifying ongoing risk.
- Being open-minded and receptive to the ideas or advice offered by the MHLT in relation to the patient's further treatment, care planning and nursing care. Patient-led care ensures that the skills of specialist practitioners are used proactively to improve the individual's experience, as opposed to a 'tick-box' approach that views mental health input as a task that needs to be completed, but has little impact on the quality of care the patient receives.

Conclusions

Mental health liaison practice has developed in the UK since the 1980s, with an increasing number of specialist nurses working in multi-professional teams based in the general hospital. Much liaison work continues to be focused on emergency settings, although the potential for mental health staff to become involved in other clinical areas is being increasingly recognised. The MHLT has an important role to play in the overall delivery of effective mental health care. The role of the team is to undertake direct clinical work with individual patients, as well as to engage in consultation activities, such as care planning and clinical supervision, as a means of supporting general hospital staff to fulfil their role in addressing psychological and mental health needs.

General hospital staff and mental health liaison practitioners both need to take responsibility for ensuring that this aspect of care is recognised by managers and health commissioners as a way of ensuring that the mental health needs of patients are given equal priority within this setting.

References

Callaghan, P., Eales, S. & Coates, T. (2002a) A review of research on the structure, process and outcome of liaison mental health services. *Journal of Psychiatric and Mental Health Nursing*, 10: 155–165.

Callaghan, P., Eales, S. & Coats, T. (2002b) Patient feedback on liaison mental health care in A&E. *Nursing Times*, 98 (21): 34–36.

Caplan, G. (1970) *The Theory and Practice of Mental Health Consultation*. New York: Basic Books.

Department of Health (1994) *Working in Partnership: the Report of the Mental Health Nursing Review Team*. London: HMSO.

Department of Health (1999) *National Service Framework for Mental Health*. London: DoH.

Department of Health (2000) *National Service Framework for Coronary Heart Disease*. London: DoH.

Department of Health (2001) *National Service Framework for Older People*. London: DoH.

Department of Health (2003) *Essence of Care: patient-focused benchmarks for clinical governance*. London: DoH.

Harrison, A. & Devey, H. (2003) Benchmarking mental health care in a general hospital. *Nursing Times*, 99 (24): 34–36.

Jones, A. (1989) Liaison consultation psychiatry: the CPN as clinical nurse specialist. *Community Psychiatric Nursing Journal*, 9 (2): 7–14.

Levenson, J.L., Hamer, R. & Rossiter, L.F. (1990) Relation of psychopathology in general medical inpatients to use and cost of services. *American Journal of Psychiatry*, 147: 1498–1503.

Lewis, C. (2004) Lost in liaison. *Health Service Journal*, April: 30–31.

Loveridge, L. & Carr, N. (1996) Advantageous liaisons. *Nursing Times*, 92 (50): 42–43.

Morriss, R. & Mayou, R. (1996) International overview of consultation-liaison psychiatry. In: E. Guthrie & F. Creed (eds) *Seminars in Liaison Psychiatry*, pp. 1–20. London: Gaskell.

National Institute for Clinical Excellence (2004a) *Improving Supportive and Palliative Care for Adults with Cancer*. London: NICE.

National Institute for Clinical Excellence (2004b) *Self-harm: the short-term physical and psychological management and secondary prevention of self-harm in primary and secondary care*. Clinical Guideline 16. London: NICE.

Peplau, H.E. (1964) Psychiatric nursing skills and the general hospital patient. *Nursing Forum*, 3 (2): 28–37.

Roberts, D. & Whitehead, L. (2002) Liaison mental health nursing: an overview of its development and current practice. In: S. Regal & D. Roberts (eds) *Mental Health Liaison*, pp. 43–63. Edinburgh: Baillière Tindall/Royal College of Nursing.

Royal College of Physicians/Royal College of Psychiatrists (1995) *The Psychological Care of Medical Patients*. London: RCP/RCPsych.

Royal College of Physicians/Royal College of Psychiatrists (2003) *The Psychological Care of Medical Patients*, 2nd edn. London: RCP/RCPsych.

Tunmore, R. (1990) The consultation liaison nurse. *Nursing*, 4 (3): 31–34.

Tunmore, R. (1994) Encouraging collaboration. *Nursing Times*, 90 (20): 66–67.

Tunmore, R. (1997) Liaison mental health nursing and mental health consultation. In: B. Thomas, S. Hardy, & P. Cutting (eds) *Mental Health Nursing: principles and practice*, pp. 207–222. London: Mosby.

Whitehead, L. & Royles, M. (2002) Deliberate self-harm: assessment and treatment interventions. In: S. Regal & D. Roberts (eds) *Mental Health Liaison*, pp. 99–125. Edinburgh: Baillière Tindall/Royal College of Nursing.

Part 2
Mental Health Care in the
General Hospital

Chapter 7
Depression and Anxiety

Chapter aims

> ## This chapter will:
>
> - describe the prevalence of depression and its relationship with physical illness
> - discuss the possible causes of depression and describe the various treatment strategies available
> - provide an overview of the concept of anxiety and its potential impact upon individuals admitted to hospital
> - identify the nurse's role in the screening and assessment of a person's mood
> - identify the core nursing interventions required when caring for a person who is depressed or anxious.

Introduction

Depression is a mood disorder that affects people in different ways and at different times of their lives. The provision of effective, sensitive and evidence-based care to those with depression can present a challenge to all health care professionals, particularly to those working in the general hospital, where prevalence is high and numerous factors militate against staff addressing mental health needs (see Chapters 1 and 2).

The presence of major depression in the general population is approximately 5%, with rates of between 2% and 4% in men, and 2% and 6% in women (Hawton & van Heeringen, 2000). Depression is a well recognised complication of numerous physical illnesses, including heart disease, stroke, cancer, neurological conditions and traumatic injury (Gelder *et al.*, 1999). Depression is missed or poorly assessed in cardiac illness and represents a significant risk factor in the morbidity and mortality associated with heart disease (Hemingway & Marmot, 2004), and as many as 16% of patients will have symptoms of a major depression when assessed seven days after a myocardial infarction (Davies *et al.*, 2004). Depression is the most common cause of long-term sick leave and accounts for more lost working days in the general population than causes such as back pain (Henderson *et al.*, 2005).

Theoretical perspectives on the causes of depression

Much research has been undertaken into the possible causes of depression. The cause of mental illness has been debated for centuries and we hear the term 'nature or nurture' used to describe the often polarised perspectives adopted by various theorists in attempting to understand the causes of mental ill health. There has been inquiry into whether illnesses such as depression are genetically determined, although contemporary thinking has moved to a multi-dimensional perspective that considers the impact of biological, psychological and social factors in the cause of depression (Table 7.1).

The role of the social environment and life experience is highlighted in the development of depression. The interaction between predisposing social and biological factors, in combination with specific precipitants can lead to a mood disorder. The association between depression and physical illnesses, such as infections, is well recognised. In order to illustrate the possible interactions between these various factors, it is important to appreciate that:

- the biological factor(s) is often the reason why the person has been admitted to hospital
- there is a complex interplay between the various predisposing and precipitating factors
- the social context or situation can often be one of the most important determinants in terms of understanding the cause of the person's depression, as well as in identifying treatment and nursing interventions.

Terms used to describe the various types of mood disorder

A number of different terms are used to classify the range of mood disorders:

- *Depressive episode* (significantly lowered mood). This may be mild, moderate or severe, and can be described as a unipolar mood disorder, in that depression is at one end of a spectrum of mood disorders.
- *Mania and hypomania* (significantly elevated mood). This is often seen as part of a bipolar mood disorder.
- *Bipolar affective disorder* (sometimes known as manic depression). This is characterised by variations or 'swings' in mood, from mania and elation at one end to depression at the other (see Chapter 10).

- *Psychotic depression*. A severe form of depressive illness with pervasive and unrelieved low mood. Delusional thinking may be present, for example, whereby the person believes that they are completely worthless and deserve to be dead, or believing that they have already died. Perceptual disturbances may also be a feature of this type of depression (see Chapter 10).
- *Organic mood disorders*. These usually occur secondary to a physical/organic abnormality (e.g. brain tumour), or metabolic disturbance (e.g. electrolyte imbalance) affecting the brain. The mood changes may appear the same or similar to depression or other psychiatric illness.

Table 7.1 Overview of the aetiology of depression.

Perspective	Commentary
Biological	Biochemical mechanisms underlying depression are complex, although the dominant hypothesis is that there is an imbalance of certain neurotransmitters within the brain. Two neurotransmitters in particular, noradrenaline and serotonin (5-hydroxy tryptamine) have been the focus of much research and subsequent development of specific medications to address this Disturbance to the neurotransmitter systems can cause alterations in sleep, appetite, motivation and pleasure, all of which are symptoms of depression Hereditary factors have been the subject of research, as depression tends to run in families Birth trauma, physical deprivation and physical illness also play a role in the development of depression
Psychological	The concept of loss is central to psychodynamic understanding of depression. Loss may be experienced as the result of bereavement, relationship break-up or redundancy Life events, even those considered to be 'positive' events, can precipitate a depressive episode: childbirth, children leaving home and job promotion all have the potential to trigger depression in vulnerable individuals Early life experiences and the impact of parental role models The development of particular cognitive schema (thinking patterns) and attribution styles are thought to be influential, e.g. core beliefs, low self-esteem and negative thinking patterns are likely to have evolved from childhood experiences
Social	Impact of gender and social class, e.g. depression is twice as common in women as in men, and more common in social classes IV and V Unemployment and employment problems, housing difficulties, financial problems, and lack of a supportive and confiding social network are all implicated There are high rates of depression in individuals who consume excessive amounts of alcohol and those who use illicit drugs

Recognising depression

When caring for patients it is important to acknowledge the links between the person's physical and psychological wellbeing. Factors involved in the development of depression may include:

- Many prescribed medications can lead to the development of depressive symptoms, for example, steroids, digoxin, beta-blockers and benzodiazepine medications (see Chapters 2, 6 and 10).
- Alcohol and illicit or non-prescription medication also needs to be considered in determining the possible cause or complicating factor. Alcohol has a depressant effect on the central nervous system, although its short-lived anxiolytic (relaxing) effect can be a factor leading to excessive consumption. All patients should be asked about alcohol use as part of a comprehensive nursing assessment (see Chapter 11).
- Pain can directly influence a person's mood. Both depression and anxiety can have an effect on an individual's perception and tolerance of pain (Davis, 2000).
- Cognitive impairment, such as poor recall and impaired concentration, can be a symptom of depression (particularly in older people) and can mask other depressive symptoms.
- It has been suggested that people prone to depression often have a negative belief (thinking) system which adversely influences their perceptions of the self (Beck, 1970). Rogers (1951) described this phenomenon as a basic mismatch between the individual's 'ideal and actual self'. This suggests that depression occurs when individuals consistently set themselves ideals and goals that they cannot hope to achieve.
- It is usual for people to experience some fluctuation in the way they feel day-to-day, sometimes hour-to-hour. This may be directly related to their environment, level of stress, how the person feels about themselves, as well as a variety of other social and interpersonal factors. The way we respond to and deal with personal challenges is largely determined by our level of confidence and our current and past ability to cope, problem-solve, make decisions and feel supported and cared about. Sometimes it is difficult to discern the difference between someone who is not coping and the person who is depressed (Table 7.2). This is particularly complicated if anxiety or stress is also present, as these symptoms are quite commonly seen together.
- Depression is twice as common in patients in the general hospital as in the rest of the population (Royal College of Physicians/Royal College of Psychiatrists, 2003). High rates of depression and other mood disorders have been reported in patients with a range of medical illnesses, in particular cardiac and neurological illness. However, many of the symptoms of depression are similar to those of the underlying physical illness, making it difficult to identify low mood in some individuals. Endicott (1984)

described a list of additional symptoms that can be used to assess the degree of depression in a person who is physically ill (Box 7.1).

■ Symptoms and severity of mood disorders may be usefully regarded as occurring across a continuum (Fig. 7.1), and individuals may experience a mood disturbance at any point on this spectrum.

Table 7.2 Possible differentiation between the person experiencing difficulty in coping and the person who is depressed.

Signs and symptoms of difficulty coping	Signs and symptoms of depression*
Low mood which responds positively when in company	Low mood
Irritability	Impaired sleep pattern
Reduced interest and sense of enjoyment	Lack of interest and enjoyment
Tendency towards emotionality	Reduced libido
Thoughts focused on the specific difficulty or problem	Alteration in appetite and weight
Mood remains responsive to external events	Tearfulness
	Expressions of hopelessness and helplessness
	Sense of no or little control over future
	Suicidal thoughts

* The above symptoms need to be consistently present for at least two weeks.

Box 7.1 Additional symptoms of depression in individuals who are medically unwell (Endicott, 1984).

■ Fearful and depressed appearance
■ Social withdrawal or reduced willingness to talk
■ Psychomotor retardation or agitation
■ Depressed mood
■ Mood does not react to environmental change or events
■ Marked reduction in interest or pleasure in most activities
■ Brooding, self pity or pessimism
■ Feelings of worthlessness, excessive or inappropriate guilt
■ Recurrent thoughts of death or suicide

Anxiety

Feelings of anxiety are a universal human experience, having evolved from the primitive 'fight or flight' response seen in all animals. Anxiety can be

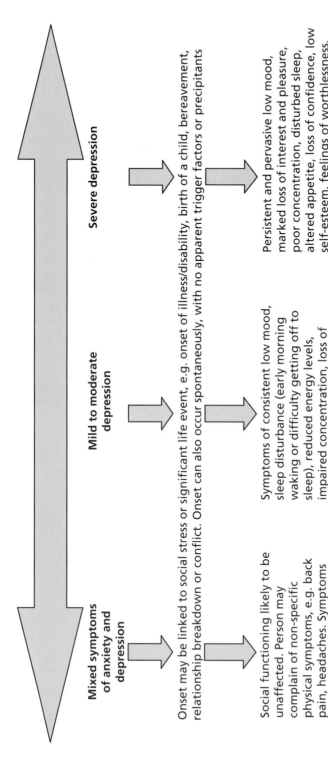

Figure 7.1 Continuum of anxiety and depression.

Table 7.3 Common signs and symptoms of anxiety.

Autonomic symptoms	Physical symptoms	Psychological symptoms
Tachycardia	Onset of tremor	Insomnia, particularly
Sweating	Muscular aches	remaining asleep
Dizziness	Shakiness	Irritability
Hot/cold spells	Lump in throat	Startles easily
Frequency of micturition	Difficulty swallowing	Feeling tense
Diarrhoea/nausea	Restlessness	Poor concentration
Paraesthesiae (pins and	Fatigue	Inability to relax
needles)	Distractible	Absence of/or reduced sense
		of humour

experienced in the absence of an apparent external threat and also as a consequence of situations and events that the individual finds unfamiliar or difficult. Events such as being admitted to hospital can trigger feelings of anxiety and can manifest in a variety of ways (Table 7.3). Anxiety affects various bodily systems and functions, but consistent among these are the often distressing physical, or somatic, symptoms.

As well as the typical symptoms described here, anxiety can also be demonstrated through behaviours such as limiting social interaction and conversation, appearing hostile or dismissive towards staff, repeatedly asking questions and seeking reassurance (see Chapter 2). Within the hospital setting a number of factors can cause anxiety (Box 7.2). Extreme or excessive anxiety and fear concerning one's health (also referred to as hypochondriasis and illness phobia) may result in a small number of individuals presenting repeatedly for tests, investigations and treatment. Such individuals do not obtain reassurance from being told that they are well, or that the results of tests were negative; as a result, this problem can become chronic. Treatment will involve

Box 7.2 Potential sources of anxiety (adapted from Pitts, 1991).

- Separation from close family, friends and confidants
- Limited amounts of information, poor quality information, lack of explanation
- Inability to access usual diversional and occupational activities
- Being in a situation that involves role reversal or loss of normal social role
- Loss of control and a sense of depersonalisation
- Possibility that procedures (e.g. surgery) will mean a loss of control, epitomised by 'being put to sleep', being cut and feeling pain

specialist assessment and specific psychological interventions, such as cognitive behavioural therapy (Kitchiner & Rogers, 2001).

It is important to remember that for most patients feelings of anxiety will be transient, and that they will respond well to appropriate explanation, reassurance and sensitive communication. For some, anxiety can become a significant problem in its own right and may require further specialist input. Treatment strategies for individuals who present with anxiety that is not self-limiting may include:

- development of breathing and relaxation techniques
- diversional activities, e.g. having a hot bath, listening to music
- development of personal coping strategies that utilise cognitive behavioural principles, e.g. recognising and addressing automatic negative thoughts and challenging these with more realistic alternatives
- short-term use of anxiolytic medication, such as diazepam, which acts by reducing emotional reactivity and somatic responses. However, because of its addictive properties, it should not be used continuously for longer than five days without a formal medical review (Hopkins, 1999)
- provision of health advice and information may be appropriate and may consist of the need to address fundamental lifestyle issues, such as:
  - □ work–home interface, e.g. addressing the impact of excessive work, amount of time spent at work, blurred boundaries between professional and personal life caused by 'bringing work home'
  - □ addressing issues around the development of a healthier lifestyle, e.g. smoking, use of alcohol, exercise
  - □ the potential benefits of developing specific strategies to manage stress, e.g. yoga, relaxation classes, aromatherapy.

Panic attacks

When a person experiences episodes of sudden, severe and uncontrollable anxiety, this is referred to as a 'panic attack'. Onset is triggered by thoughts of dread and fear, which can involve new or previously stressful situations, for example, social activities such as shopping. Certain situations can act as triggers to a panic attack, such as visiting the dentist or coming into hospital. A panic attack is characterised by the following:

(1) thinking that something awful is about to happen, for example, suffering a heart attack and then dying
(2) somatic symptoms then act as reinforcement to the underlying thoughts and are likely to include palpitations, sweating, parasthesiae and hyperventilation.

Phobias

Phobias are irrational fears that are out of proportion to the actual threat posed to the individual (Russell, 1999) and are classified as follows:

- *Agoraphobia*. This is characterised by avoidance of specific places or situations, triggered by the belief that the person will experience an overwhelming sense of anxiety and panic. Such feelings may lead to marked social disability and may include situations such as being in shops and supermarkets, using public transport and visiting hospital.
- *Social phobia*. This is characterised by excessive performance anxiety regarding situations such as talking in front of others, public speaking and ordering food in restaurants.
- *Specific phobias*. These involve marked anxiety and feelings of panic triggered by discrete situations. Examples may include a phobia of certain animals, such as rodents or snakes; fear of attending the dentist; fear of needles and injections in medical situations.

Often the person will become anxious and fearful in the specific situations described above, while other aspects of their life remain relatively unaffected, provided that they avoid the object, situation or event that triggers it. In order to minimise feelings of anxiety, the individual avoids or limits exposure to the situation that triggers the response. For many, such avoidance has little impact on their life and social functioning, but in some cases the avoidance behaviour becomes extreme and disabling. The person may be fully aware that the fear or phobia is irrational, but remain unable to overcome it, despite explanation and logical persuasion. Phobias are relatively common; however, treatment for specific phobias, which severely restrict the person's life style, will usually involve specialist psychological intervention.

Assessment

Developing an understanding of the person's mood is a core aspect of an holistic nursing assessment, and to ensure that this is afforded appropriate attention, an effective assessment framework needs to be in place (Table 7.4).

There is a role for the use of standardised screening tools and a number have been used in physical care settings, with evidence that they can provide a useful adjunct to the assessment process (Bowling, 2001). It is important to remember that they are not designed as diagnostic instruments and data obtained should be used to enhance the assessment, rather than being the sole source of information used to decide on treatment. Specific screening tools include:

- *General Health Questionnaire* (GHQ). A commonly used scale of psychiatric morbidity, which focuses on detecting anxiety and depression. It is used across a wide range of clinical settings and is designed for self-completion.

Table 7.4 Key information required when assessing mood.

Aspect of assessment	Key information
Patient's subjective account	Note whether: Tearful Mood is 'flat' or blunt Exhibits reduced social interaction and communication that is not explained by physical impairment or environment
Pathological factors	Note whether the patient may be predisposed to becoming depressed or anxious because of: Side effects or consequences of medical treatments, e.g. medication, radiotherapy Cerebral damage, e.g. following stroke, head injury Pre-existing medical or other physical health problems
Psychological factors	Note potential or actual impact of: History of mood or other psychiatric disorder (particularly depression or anxiety) Recent significant life events, e.g. bereavement, childbirth, relationship problems
Physical factors	Note potential or actual impact of: Physical deficits or problems as a result of illness or injury, e.g. aphasia, immobility, degree of physical dependence
Social factors	Note potential or actual impact of: Employment, e.g. role within family unit, whether patient is the main source of family income Housing Financial worries or concerns
Interpersonal factors	Note potential or actual impact of: Input from partner/significant other, family members, friends Pre-morbid relationship, e.g. avoid making assumptions about the role of the person's partner in providing ongoing care and support; involve significant other in discussions regarding his or her level of input and involvement in the recovery and rehabilitation process

Several versions exist (including the GHQ 28 and GHQ 30) and it has evaluated well in tests of validity, reliability and sensitivity (Goldberg & Williams, 1988).

- *Hospital Anxiety and Depression Scale* (HADS). A self-completion questionnaire designed to detect anxiety and depression in individuals with physical illness. The depression items have been designed to ensure that they do not relate to the symptoms of physical illness or injury, making it more sensitive in detecting depression in general hospital patients. It consists of 14 items, seven for anxiety and seven for depression, and requires yes/no responses (Zigmond & Snaith, 1983).

- *Beck's Depression Inventory* (BDI). A self-rating questionnaire that is based on the person's subjective experience. The full version has 21 items and a modified version made up of 13 items has also been developed. Both stress the cognitive symptoms of depression. The patient selects the responses that best fit how they have been feeling during the past week. Good reliability and validity has been reported, although most studies have evaluated its use in psychiatric populations, as opposed to its use in individuals with physical illness. Despite this, it is also used with patients who have a physical illness (Lustman, 1997).
- *Geriatric Depression Scale* (GDS). The full version contains 30 items, although a shorter version containing 15 items also exists. It can be completed by the patient and also be administered by the nurse. The questionnaire consists of yes/no responses to questions that focus on the person's subjective experience of depression (Yesavage *et al.*, 1983).

Treatment strategies for depression

This section provides a summary of the treatment strategies for depression.

Physical treatments

Antidepressant medication is one of the major treatments for depression and has been available since the 1950s. The biochemical mechanisms underlying depression are complex, but appear to be linked to either an imbalance or a deficiency of specific neurotransmitters, particularly noradrenaline and serotonin (5-HT). Tricyclic antidepressants (TCAs) were the first to be discovered, followed by selective serotonin reuptake inhibitors (SSRIs) in the late 1980s. Despite their extensive use, their exact mode of action is not fully understood, although treatment is aimed at restoring the balance of neuro-regulating amines by blocking the uptake (TCAs) or reuptake (SSRIs) in the brain.

Another group of drugs, known as monoamine oxidase inhibitors (MAOIs), works by inhibiting the breakdown of neurotransmitters by enzymes such as amine oxidase (Hopkins, 1999). There are various types of antidepressant (Table 7.5), and the choice of which one is used will be influenced by the following:

- Prescriber's experience and personal choice.
- Side effect profile – groups of antidepressants have specific side effect profiles; for example, TCAs are more likely to cause drowsiness than SSRIs.
- Patient's previous history of depression and treatment.
- Presence, or otherwise, of medical illness.
- Safety profile of the medication in overdose – it is common for people suffering from depression to contemplate suicide. Individuals considered at high suicide risk should not be prescribed antidepressants with a high toxicity in overdose (see Chapter 8).
- Patient preference.

Table 7.5 Major antidepressants.*

Class	Examples	Notes
Tricyclic antidepressants (TCAs)	Amitriptyline Clomipramine Doxepin Lofepramine	Significant side effect profile, due to anticholinergic effects, e.g. dry mouth, drowsiness and sedation, palpitations, dizziness, blurred vision, constipation, sexual dysfunction, weight gain, postural hypotension Cardio-toxic – should be avoided in patients with cardiac disease. Particularly cardio-toxic in overdose High fatality rate in overdose – should not be prescribed to those considered at high risk of suicide
Selective noradrenaline reuptake inhibitors (SNRIs) and selective serotonin reuptake inhibitors (SSRIs)	Venlafaxine Citalopram Fluvoxamine Fluoxetine Paroxetine Sertraline	Fewer cholinergic side effects than TCAs Side effects include headache, insomnia, nausea, subjective feelings of anxiety and nervousness, sexual dysfunction Overall, less toxic than TCAs and safer in overdose Should not be used as first line treatment in patients with mild to moderate depression SNRIs should only be prescribed by specialist mental health clinicians (NICE, 2004)
Noradrenaline reuptake inhibitors (NaRIs)	Reboxetine Mirtazapine	Generally well tolerated antidepressants Less likely to be associated with the side effects of agitation, anxiety and insomnia that are linked with SSRIs
Monoamine oxidase inhibitors (MAOIs)	Selegiline Isocarboxazid	Usually prescribed by specialists and used for the treatment of depression that has failed to respond to first line treatments Inhibits the metabolism of tyramine (found in certain foods, such as cheese, red meat and yeast extract). Increased tyramine can lead to hypertension, over activity and delirium; therefore, patients should be advised to avoid the foods listed above At least two weeks must elapse between discontinuing MAOIs and treatment with another antidepressant

* Refer to latest edition of the *British National Formulary (BNF)* before prescription or administration.

There is limited difference in the overall efficacy of various antidepressants, although some are better tolerated, primarily due to the presence or otherwise of specific side effects. Patients are less likely to stop taking SSRIs/SNRIs than TCAs, because of their lower side effect profile. Consensus is that antidepressants should not be used as a first line treatment in people with mild to moderate depression, as the risk–benefit ratio is poor (National Institute for Clinical Excellence (NICE), 2004). Whenever antidepressants are prescribed, treatment should be at the correct therapeutic dose and should be continued for a minimum of six months once the original symptoms have resolved (Healey, 2002).

Electroconvulsive therapy (ECT) consists of passing an electrical current through the brain, following the administration of a general anaesthetic. The exact mode of action is unclear, although it is thought that the current stimulates dopanergic pathways, causing an increase in the neurotransmitter and its metabolites, resulting in a rapid antidepressant effect (Porter & Ferrier, 1999). Side effects of ECT include headache, confusion and short-term memory loss. Although well established, ECT remains a controversial treatment and guidance recommends that its use be confined to cases of severe depression, when all other forms of treatment have failed to produce an elevation in mood (NICE, 2003).

Psychological treatments

A number of psychological treatments (Moore & McLaughlin, 2003) are available for use in depression (Table 7.6), including counselling, cognitive behavioural therapy, problem-solving and systemic family therapy. In order to deliver these, nurses require specific training and supervision. In general, specialist therapy is limited, although there are examples of non-mental health nurses developing specific elements of therapies such as cognitive behavioural therapy and problem-solving, and providing this as part of a holistic approach to care for people with physical illness (Edwards & Feber, 2003; Grimmer et al., 2004).

Newer methods of delivering cognitive behavioural therapy have been developed, primarily as a means of addressing the limited access to specialist therapists. Cognitive behavioural therapy and a number of derivatives are available as computerised packages, and can be accessed by patients directly, or in collaboration with health staff, as CD-ROMs and internet-based options (Illman, 2004).

Combination of physical and psychological treatments

Given the multi-factorial nature of depression, and the complex interplay of predisposing and precipitating factors, a treatment approach that combines both physical and psychological treatments is likely to be more effective in alleviating the symptoms (World Health Organization, 2000). When the person is cared for within the general hospital, there is an important role for both types of intervention.

Table 7.6 Overview of the main psychological treatments for depression.

Treatment	Comments
Counselling or interpersonal psychotherapy	Non-specific talking therapy, usually based on humanistic principles and using the skills of active listening, warmth and empathy. Limited evidence regarding its efficacy as a treatment for depression, although nurses are increasingly being encouraged to develop counselling skills for use in practice (Freshwater, 2003)
Cognitive behavioural therapy	Specific talking therapy focusing on two elements thought to have a major influence on the development and experience of depression, namely cognition (thoughts) and behaviour (actions). The aim is to assist the person to recognise the link between negative and unhelpful thoughts (such as irrational beliefs) and the behaviours that are associated with them. Has been evaluated positively as a treatment for depression and it is recommended that it be more widely available throughout the NHS (NICE, 2002). One American study has suggested that cognitive behavioural therapy is as effective as medication in the treatment of moderate to severe depression (DeRubeis et al., 2005). Requires specialist training, although it is possible for non-mental health nurses to utilise cognitive and behavioural techniques as part of routine nursing care (Edwards & Feber, 2003)
Problem-solving	Focused talking therapy that assists the person to identify the current social, health or interpersonal problems in order of impact and priority in their life. With support and guidance from the therapist, the individual identifies possible solutions to the problems and works on strategies to implement these. When delivered by suitably trained staff, there is evidence as to its effectiveness in physical care settings (Strong et al., 2004)
Systemic family therapy	Family therapy aims to work alongside patients and their families to explore the ways that problems, illness, disability and disease affect them and others within the context of everyday life. The focus of such a therapeutic approach is to view the patient and the family as a unit functioning as a whole system. There is evidence as to its effectiveness in the management of depression (Leff et al., 2000)

Planning care for the person who is depressed or anxious

Caring for the person who is depressed or anxious requires the practitioner to focus on:

- effective use of interpersonal skills
- responding and attending to specific biological, psychological and social needs.

Use of interpersonal skills

Individuals who are depressed are likely to experience a range of negative emotions, including feelings of hopelessness, helplessness, frustration and negativity. Many nurses find dealing with such feelings difficult, and within a busy clinical environment it can be easy to negate the person's distress either by focusing on practical, physically-orientated tasks or by limiting face-to-face contact. Effective use of self can be demonstrated by developing skills such as active listening, responding to patient cues, showing warmth, interest and empathy, and the appropriate use of touch. While it is necessary to offer a sense of hope, it is important to avoid giving overly prescriptive advice or false reassurance. Although well meaning, statements such as, 'Don't worry, everything will be all right', are likely to increase the person's sense of distress and feelings of disempowerment.

Questions can assist in the identification of how the person is feeling as well as highlight specific concerns, worries and problems that may be acting as psychological reinforcements for depressive thoughts and feelings. Closed questions require a yes or no response, and are useful for eliciting or confirming factual information. Examples include 'Do you feel more depressed than last week?' and 'Has your sleep pattern been disturbed?' Although useful, such questions do not allow for the exploration of thoughts and feelings and, if used excessively, may impart a lack of interest.

The use of open questions such as, 'How are you feeling?' and 'What is it that is making you feel so anxious?' create opportunities to explore what it is that may be influencing the person's current emotional state. Often such feelings are triggered and maintained by concern over relatively simple or straightforward issues, such as practical tasks, including transport, pets and visiting times. More serious concerns may also be brought to the fore, such as thoughts of self-harm or suicide, degree of pain and discomfort, and the effect of specific treatments such as side effects of medication.

Responding to the person's care needs

Nursing responses will need to ensure that the person receives the appropriate level of care and support (Table 7.7), which address:

- *Communication*. Depression and anxiety both impair the person's ability to communicate effectively. Common difficulties include withdrawing from routine social interaction, isolation and difficulty in expressing feelings. The ability of the nurse to demonstrate empathy, warmth and hope are core interpersonal skills that will underpin all other nursing assessment and intervention activity.
- *Maintaining a safe environment*. All depressed patients are likely to have experienced thoughts of self-harm or suicide. Identification of risk and the implementation of appropriate strategies to manage specific risks are key nursing responsibilities (see Chapter 8).

Table 7.7 Nursing assessment and interventions for the person who is depressed.

Intervention	Rationale
Include assessment and evaluation of mood within initial nursing assessment processes	Provides baseline against which to measure changes to mood during hospital stay
Utilise non-judgemental approach and active listening skills when communicating with the person	Demonstrates acceptance, value, warmth and empathy. All of these factors can have a positive therapeutic effect on the person's mood and self-esteem
Provide protected time in order to engage the person in a discussion regarding their current thoughts and feelings	Demonstrates acceptance and reinforces holistic care
Identify specific symptoms of depression associated with their physical illness, or as a result of current treatments, e.g. side effects of medication	Certain depressive symptoms can be a direct consequence of the underlying physical illness/injury, or a consequence of prescribed medical treatments
Identify whether there are any pre-existing or related factors contributing to apparent depressive feelings or behaviour, e.g. interpersonal difficulties, financial worries, recent bereavement	Assists in the screening and diagnosis of depression in patients admitted to hospital
If depression is suspected, encourage and support the person in completing an appropriate screening tool	Provides standardised baseline against which to measure changes to mood during hospital stay
Identify whether the person has any suicidal and/or self-harming thoughts. If self-harming or suicidal thoughts are present, complete suicide risk screen (see Chapter 8)	Depression is associated with an increased risk of self-harm and suicide
Explain that depressive feelings are a common consequence of physical illness and hospital admission	Utilising time to discuss thoughts and feelings can assist in normalising the individual's experience
Discuss with the multi-disciplinary team any concerns regarding the patient's mood	Demonstrates effective team working and collaboration. Effective communication helps ensure appropriate care and can assist in the reduction of risk
If antidepressant medication is indicated, ensure that it is administered as prescribed	Ensures that appropriate treatment is commenced as soon as possible
Explain that antidepressant medication can take up to three weeks before demonstrating a positive therapeutic effect	Concordance and collaboration is improved if the person is aware of all the facts and options regarding the use of antidepressants

Table 7.7 (*Cont'd*)

Intervention	Rationale
Monitor patient response to both therapeutic and side effects of any antidepressant medication prescribed	Provides valuable information about the person's response to treatment
Observe and record details of the person's verbal and non-verbal behaviour, e.g. anger, impulsivity, irritability, motor retardation, dietary and fluid intake	Ensures that the appropriate level of care is initiated, e.g. recovery from depression is enhanced if adequate nutrition, hydration and physical activity are maintained
If concerned over the person's mood or if deterioration continues, consider referral to mental health liaison staff for specialist advice and assessment (see Chapter 6)	Mental health liaison staff can assist in treatment and care. Ensures specialist follow up and onward referral is arranged, if appropriate

- *Alleviating low mood.* Skilled nursing care is an intervention in its own right and no nurse should underestimate the impact this can have. Feeling valued and cared for are both likely to have a positive effect on the individual's self-esteem and mood.
- *Physical.* Poor physical health can be a precipitant for depression, but depression can also have a detrimental effect on physical wellbeing and can impair recovery and rehabilitation (Rinomhota & Marshall, 2000). Common physical problems associated with depression and anxiety include:
  □ impaired appetite – either loss of appetite (anorexia), or increased food intake as a reaction to stress
  □ disturbed sleep – may present as either insomnia or hypersomnia (excessive sleeping)
  □ loss of interest in appearance – leading to difficulty in washing, dressing and maintaining personal hygiene
  □ increased or decreased physical activity – motor retardation may be a feature of severe depression, and increased activity, agitation and restlessness can be features of marked anxiety states.

Conclusions

Depression and anxiety are common problems and are seen frequently in patients within the general hospital. Both depression and anxiety are common complications of a range of physically based illnesses, although they are both issues that health professionals often fail to recognise and treat adequately. Untreated depression remains a major factor in relation to problems such as delayed hospital discharge, slowed recovery and rehabilitation, and failed community care. The multi-factorial causes of depression mean that it is a problem that requires the practitioner to adopt a holistic perspective when assessing and caring for the person who is experiencing a low mood. The key factors are the need to raise the awareness of non-mental health staff to these problems, as well as for them to play an active role in the care and treatment of the depressed person.

References

Beck, A.T. (1970) *Depression: causes and treatment*. Philadelphia: University of Pennsylvania Press.

Bowling, A. (2001) *Measuring Disease*, 2nd edn., pp. 74–98. Buckingham: Open University Press.

Davies, S.J.C., Jackson, P.R. & Potokar, J. (2004) Treatment of anxiety and depressive disorders in patients with cardiovascular disease. *British Medical Journal*, 328: 939–943.

Davis, B. (2000) *Caring For People in Pain*. London: Routledge.

DeRubeis, R.J., Hollon, S.D. & Amsterdam, J.D. (2005) Cognitive therapy vs medications in the treatment of moderate to severe depression. *Archives of General Psychiatry*, 62: 409–416.

Edwards, M. & Feber, T. (2003) Working with anxiety in cancer: psycho-oncological care. *Cancer Nursing Practice*, 2 (1): 19–26.

Endicott, J. (1984) Measurement of depression in outpatients with cancer. *Cancer*, 53 (10): 2243–2249.

Freshwater, D. (2003) *Counselling Skills for Nurses, Midwives and Health Visitors*. Maidenhead: Open University Press.

Gelder, M., Mayou, R. & Geddes, J. (1999) *Psychiatry*, 2nd edn. Oxford: Oxford University Press.

Goldberg, D.P. & Williams, P. (1988) *A User's Guide to the General Health Questionnaire*. Windsor: NFER-Nelson.

Grimmer, L., Atterbury, C. & Keidan, J. (2004) Monitoring quality of life in patients with haematological malignancies. *Cancer Nursing Practice*, 3 (7): 24–30.

Hawton, K. & van Heeringen, K. (2000) *The International Handbook of Suicide and Attempted Suicide*. Chichester: John Wiley & Sons.

Healey, D. (2002) *Psychiatric Drugs Explained*. Edinburgh: Churchill Livingstone.

Hemingway, H. & Marmot, M. (2004) Psychosocial factors in the aetiology and prognosis of coronary heart disease: systematic review of prospective cohort studies. *British Medical Journal*, 318: 1460–1467.

Henderson, M., Glozier, N. & Holland-Elliott, K. (2005) Long term sickness absence. *British Medical Journal*, 330: 802–803.

Hopkins, S.J. (1999) *Drugs and Pharmacology for Nurses*, 13th edn. Edinburgh: Churchill Livingstone.

Illman, J. (2004) Switching on to cognitive therapy. *Nursing Standard*, 19 (12): 16–17.

Kitchiner, N. & Rogers, P. (2001) Health anxiety (hypochondriasis; illness phobia): nature, assessment and treatment. *Mental Health Practice*, 4 (8): 32–38.

Leff, J., Vearnals, S. & Wolff, G. (2000) The London depression intervention trial. *British Journal of Psychiatry*, 177 (2): 95–100.

Lustman, P. (1997) Screening for depression in diabetes using the Beck Depression Inventory. *Psychosomatic Medicine*, 59 (1): 24–31.

Moore, K. & McLaughlin, D. (2003) Depression: the challenge for all healthcare professionals. *Nursing Standard*, 17 (26): 45–52.

National Institute for Clinical Excellence (2002) *Computerised Cognitive Behavioural Therapy for Anxiety and Depression*. London: NICE.

National Institute for Clinical Excellence (2003) *Guidance on the Use of Electroconvulsive Therapy*. London: NICE.

National Institute for Clinical Excellence (2004) *Guidelines to Improve the Treatment and Care of People with Depression and Anxiety*. London: NICE.

Pitts, M. (1991) The experience of treatment. In: M. Pitts & K. Phillips (eds.) *The Psychology of Health*. London: Routledge.

Porter, R. & Ferrier, N. (1999) Emergency treatment of depression. *Advances in Psychiatric Treatment*, 5: 3–10.

Rinomhota, A.S. & Marshall, P. (2000) *Biological Aspects of Mental Health Nursing*. Edinburgh: Churchill Livingstone.

Rogers, C. (1951) *Client Centred Therapy*. Boston: Houghton Mifflin.

Royal College of Physicians/Royal College of Psychiatrists (2003) *The Psychological Care of Medical Patients*, 2nd edn. London: RCP/RCPsych.

Russell, G. (1999) *Essential Psychology for Nurses and Other Health Professionals*. London: Routledge.

Strong, V., Sharpe, M. & Cull, A. (2004) Can oncology nurses treat depression? A pilot project. *Journal of Advanced Nursing*, 46 (5): 542–548.

World Health Organization (2000) *WHO Guide to Mental Health in Primary Care*. London: Royal Society of Medicine Press.

Yesavage, J., Brink, T. & Rose, T. (1983) Geriatric Depression Scale (GDS): recent evidence and development of a shorter version. *Journal of Psychiatric Research*, 17: 37–49.

Zigmond, A.S. & Snaith, R.P. (1983) The Hospital Anxiety and Depression Scale. *Acta Psychiatrica Scandinavica*, 67: 361–370.

Chapter 8
Self-harm and Suicide Prevention

Chapter aims

This chapter will:

- explore the descriptions and terminology used in relation to self-harm and self-harming behaviour
- describe the incidence, precipitants and motivations relating to self-harming behaviour
- discuss nurses' perceptions of self-harming behaviour and the impact that staff attitudes can have upon the person when admitted following an episode of self-harm
- identify the role of the non-specialist nurse in the assessment of suicide risk
- describe the role of the general hospital nurse in the treatment and care of the person who has self-harmed
- describe the components of effective care planning for the person who has self-harmed.

Introduction

Self-harm is one of the most common reasons for admission to and attendance at hospital (Hawton & Fagg, 1992), yet it is also one of the clinical problems that health care staff lack confidence in treating. Many patients describe unhelpful and at times uncaring responses from staff when attending hospital, while staff often find caring for individuals who self-harm challenging and unrewarding. This chapter explores some of the motivations for self-harming behaviour, as well as addressing the role of the general hospital nurse in providing safe and effective care for the person who has engaged in self-harm.

A quarter of UK suicides are preceded by hospital attendance as a result of self-harm (Gairin *et al.*, 2003), although significant numbers of these individuals may not receive a specialist psychosocial assessment prior to discharge home (Horrocks *et al.*, 2003). There is a relationship between self-harm and suicide, but identifying those individuals who are at the greatest risk is a challenging and complex task. It is also a task that may be made harder by the fact that when a person is admitted to, or attends hospital, the underlying reasons for the act may be missed due to the urgency to treat the physical injury and symptoms (Roberts, 1996).

Terminology

The term 'self-harm' is a generic phrase used to describe a wide range of self-injurious behaviours, including self-poisoning (overdose), deliberately cutting the body, jumping from a height, asphyxiation from motor gas, head banging, burning and scalding, hair pulling, and excessive use of substances such as alcohol and illicit drugs. However, these behaviours do not help us understand the motivations behind the act, something that is particularly important given the relationship between self-harm and suicide. Self-harming behaviour alone does not necessarily confirm that the person wanted to die, or that they will remain suicidal following the act. In order to clarify this, it is helpful to consider self-harm as an umbrella term, with three distinct, but overlapping, sub-groups of self-injurious behaviour (Fig. 8.1). It is important to remember, however, that the motivations will often overlap and individuals can present with characteristics from each sub-category.

Although it is important to try to establish what the underlying motivations were, this is not always obvious or easy. What is clear is that it is only the minority of self-harming presentations that are motivated by a clear, unequivocal and ongoing desire to be dead; the majority being acts that occur in 'conditions of emotional turmoil' (Kerkhof, 2000), and are often impulsive responses to some form of interpersonal crisis. Self-harm is often an extreme response to a personal crisis, and while the crisis continues the person may remain at increased risk of suicide. This is one of the reasons why a specialist assessment by mental health staff is an important component of a comprehensive plan of care.

Incidence of self-harming and suicidal behaviour

Because of the nature of self-harm, it is difficult to be precise as to its frequency. Much self-harm remains hidden, taking place in private and not coming to the attention of health and social care professionals. Overall, rates of self-harm in the UK are among the highest in Europe, accounting for approximately 150 000 hospital attendances annually (Richardson, 2004).

There are approximately 4500 suicides every year in England, this being the commonest cause of death in young men under 35 (Department of Health

Physical self-injury

Common motivating factors

- Feelings of frustration, anger, low self-esteem
- Means of communicating distress
- Means of managing and coping with negative feelings, often those produced as a result of difficult or problematic interpersonal communication
- Response to underlying beliefs and a habitual negative coping strategy
- Rarely are actions motivated by suicidal intent

Typical behaviours and presentation

- Cutting, scratching and burning the skin – most frequently arms and legs
- May present as withdrawn, uncommunicative and passive following injury

Impulsive self-harm

Common motivating factors

- Overwhelming sense of ambivalence – simultaneous beliefs about two opposing actions. For example, on the one hand wanting to die, but on the other wanting to live as long as the emotional pain would disappear
- Impulsive action often linked to use of alcohol immediately beforehand
- Short-lived perception that death is the only solution to current crisis
- Often precipitated by some form of interpersonal crisis, e.g. argument with partner/significant other

Typical behaviours and presentation

- Overdose of medication the most common form of self-harm
- Impulsive decision to end life
- Likely to seek help after taking the overdose, such as calling an ambulance
- Expressions of subsequent regret and embarrassment at actions afterwards

Attempted suicide

Common motivating factors

- Suicidal thoughts consistently present over a period of weeks, months or years
- Well thought through and considered plan to end life
- Unable to contemplate life continuing
- Unshakable belief that others 'will be better off without me'
- Feelings of ongoing hopelessness present

Typical behaviours and presentation

- Likely to have taken precautions against discovery – may only have come to the attention of others due to miscalculation or un-envisaged interruption by another person
- More likely to have used a violent method to harm self, e.g. hanging and firearms
- Likely to express regret that actions failed to result in death

Figure 8.1 Common forms of self-harming behaviour and their presentations.

Table 8.1 The most common methods people use to harm themselves (DoH, 2003b).

Method	Rate (%)
Self-poisoning (overdose)	90
Cutting and lacerations	9
Other	1

Table 8.2 The most common ways in which people kill themselves (DoH, 2003b).

Method	Rate (%)
Males	
Hanging	42
Self-poisoning	26
Other	22
Jumping	5
Motor gas	5
Females	
Self-poisoning	48
Hanging	27
Other	15
Jumping	7
Motor gas	3

(DoH), 2003b). Suicide rates are higher in males of all ages, with the peak incidence being between the ages of 19 and 34 years. Overall, the suicide rate has fallen during the past 20 years, with the exception of this age group.

Overdose of medication is the most common way in which people harm themselves, although there are variations between the methods chosen, as well as gender differences in the means of suicide (Tables 8.1 and 8.2). Non-fatal self-harm, in particular self-inflicted lacerations, is more common in females than males, although rates are rising in men.

The risk of suicide is higher in people who have previously self-harmed. One per cent of people will kill themselves in the 12 months following self-harm, increasing to 3% in the subsequent five years (Hawton *et al.*, 1997). Experiencing a mental illness increases the person's risk of suicide (Table 8.3), with depression being the most common mental disorder associated with both suicide and self-harm (Gelder *et al.*, 1999).

The suicide rate is higher among people who suffer from various physical illnesses (Box 8.1), particularly those that are associated with painful symptoms, have long-term lifestyle implications and are likely to be terminal (Harris & Barraclough, 1994).

Table 8.3 Percentage of people suffering from a mental illness and committing suicide (Hawton & van Heeringen, 2000).

	Percentage suffering from a mental illness at the time of death
Depression	50
Schizophrenia	10
Substance abuse	25
Personality disorder	31

Box 8.1 Physical illness associated with an increased risk of suicide (Stenager & Stenager, 2000).

- HIV and AIDS
- Huntingdon's disease
- Cancer
- Multiple sclerosis
- Peptic ulcer
- Renal disease
- Spinal cord injuries
- Diabetes
- Epilepsy
- Systemic lupus erythematosus

'Causes' of self-harming behaviour

There is a wide variation in the types of self-harming behaviour and their motivations (see Fig. 8.1), and there is limited research into the triggers and precipitants to such acts. What is clear is that each patient must be seen and assessed as an individual, with unique reasons for engaging in self-harm. Understanding the reasons behind the self-harm will be enhanced by a thorough assessment of the predisposing factors, precipitants and motivations. It is vital to remember that the motivations can only be fully evaluated following a specialist psychosocial assessment. Judgements relating to why the person has self-harmed and what the subsequent risk of suicide is cannot be made simply by considering the method alone.

For some individuals self-harm will have been motivated by a wish, however fleetingly, to die. However, this is not always the case, even when the person might appear to have made a serious attempt to die. In a study of individuals admitted following self-harm, a third wanted to die at the time of the act, a quarter did not want to die and a third were ambivalent about whether they lived or died (Hawton *et al.*, 1996).

The precipitating factors may have built up over a period of weeks or months, but some form of interpersonal conflict or crisis often triggers the act. Significant numbers of patients will be intoxicated with alcohol or a combination of alcohol and other substances. However, it is likely that there is a complex interplay of interpersonal, psychological and social factors that trigger the action, and in many instances the patient may describe the final trigger as being something that is relatively minor or insignificant. A summary of the precipitating, predisposing and maintaining factors is provided in Table 8.4.

Table 8.4 Predisposing, precipitating and maintaining factors relating to self-harm and suicide.

	Predisposing	**Precipitating**	**Maintaining**
Social	Family history of self-harm and suicide Abuse as a child, particularly sexual abuse Homelessness Physical illness	Entering care Parents divorcing Bereavement Rape and sexual assault Unplanned/ unwanted pregnancy Significant financial problems Lack of availability of specialist help for high risk individuals	Being bullied Unresolved housing, employment and financial problems Ready availability of potentially lethal means of self-harm, e.g. over-the-counter analgesics
Psychological	Family history of mental illness Reduced ability to regulate emotions Poor impulse control Low self-esteem	Mental illness Excessive alcohol Illicit drug use	Intoxication with alcohol and/or illicit drugs Cognitive problems, e.g. negative thinking, thoughts of worthlessness, hopelessness about the future Believing that their distress or problems are not being taken seriously by others
Interpersonal	Conflict between parents Lack of supportive, close relationship(s) Poor interpersonal problem-solving	Perceived stressful situations involving others Relationship breakdown Argument/verbal conflict with partner or significant other	Unresolved conflict with parents Continuing negative experiences of care Ongoing difficulty in communicating feelings

Attitudes

Caring for a person who has self-harmed or who has attempted suicide can be challenging to professionals. Such behaviour often evokes strong personal and professional feelings, with many practitioners identifying that caring for this group of patients is unrewarding and deskilling (Perego, 1999). Within a busy medical or emergency unit staff will be expected to care for people with a wide variety of physical health care needs and because of this, it can often feel difficult to view people who have self-harmed with the same degree of professional objectivity as patients with other problems. This may result in these patients being seen as 'time-wasters', or as somehow less deserving of treatment and care than patients with other clinical problems (Lynn, 1998; Murray, 1998).

Staff may view self-harming behaviour as a form of 'attention-seeking', and in order to avoid reinforcing such behaviour, will often distance themselves emotionally from the patient. Such attitudes are often symbolised by actions such as limiting communication, keeping the patient waiting, avoiding the person and the adoption of a sarcastic or patronising manner. Attitudes to people who have self-harmed are often negative, with both professionals and patients reporting high levels of dissatisfaction regarding their experience of care (Hemmings, 1999; Pembroke, 2000). Such attitudes will have a negative effect on both the nurse's ability to plan patient-focused care and the patient's experience of seeking help and treatment (Box 8.2).

Because self-harm is often an overt expression of psychological and emotional distress, staff may tend to avoid these patients, preferring instead to care for people with more concrete and understandable physical health problems (Hunt, 1993). Many non-mental health nurses view patients with psychiatric problems as 'unpopular' and unrewarding to care for (Brinn, 2000; James, 2004). Common feelings identified by staff include those of frustration, negativity, hopelessness, fear and anger, they also feel unsupported.

Box 8.2 The potential impact of negative attitudes towards individuals who have self-harmed.

Reinforces stereotypical and misinformed beliefs about the nature of self-harm and those who engage in it

Maintains a spiral of negative feelings and expectations among both staff and patients

Reduces the ability to view the patient and his or her problems as unique

Interferes with the ability of staff to make effective judgements regarding the assessment of risk, the planning of care and the identification of ongoing need

Increases the likelihood of patients feeling frustrated and dissatisfied with their care and treatment

Table 8.5 Common feelings experienced by patients and professionals in relation to self-harm.

Patients	Professionals
Embarrassment	Negative
Shame	Deskilled
Anger	Frustration
Helplessness	Anger
Disempowerment	Exasperation
Ignored	Challenged
Frustration	Hopelessness
Not cared for	Stressed
Self-dislike	
Derealisation – a feeling that people, events or surroundings have changed and are unreal.	

Paradoxically, such feelings often mirror what the person who has self-harmed is experiencing (Babiker & Arnold, 1997; Hopkins, 2002), and it can be useful for staff to consider their own feelings in relation to those described by patients (Table 8.5).

It is important that staff make every effort to gain insight into and acknowledge the feelings that are generated when caring for the person who has self-harmed or attempted suicide. The use of guided reflection through clinical supervision sessions and staff support groups can be a useful way of dealing with these feelings. Such activity will reduce the likelihood of patients experiencing negative communication and interactions from staff and should be considered as an essential component of practice when caring for a person who repeatedly attends hospital as a result of self-harm.

Risk assessment

All patients who present following self-harm should receive a specialist psychosocial assessment from a mental health professional (National Institute for Clinical Excellence, 2004), although it is acknowledged that significant numbers leave hospital without such an assessment. This may be for a number of reasons, including patient refusal, excessive waiting times, or a decision to discharge the person without making a referral to mental health staff. However, in order to make a decision as to whether it is appropriate to discharge the person without a specialist assessment, it is important that general hospital staff undertake a baseline suicide risk assessment. Such a decision should be based on an evaluation of all the relevant risk characteristics, as well as the individual circumstances and precipitants relating to the act.

Risk assessment is an important, but often-neglected aspect of care (Horrocks *et al.*, 2003). It is also one of the elements of care that many general hospital nurses lack the confidence and skill to address, describing various forms of avoidance behaviour and negative labelling (Perego, 1999). National guidance has long recommended that every general hospital have effective arrangements in place for the assessment and treatment of individuals admitted following self-harm (DHSS, 1984). More recently, the publication *Essence of Care* (DoH, 2003a) seeks to ensure that individuals with mental health needs are cared for in a safe and holistic way in the general hospital.

Negative attitudes can lead to minimising of the act by staff, which in turn may mean that formal attempts to assess the person's level of risk are overlooked or avoided. However, risk assessment is important because:

■ a significant number of individuals may not wait for, or may refuse, a specialist psychosocial assessment by mental health staff (Greenwood & Bradley, 1997)
■ it will allow staff to identify the priorities for immediate clinical management, plan the person's ongoing care and effectively manage any risk issues or behaviours that he or she may display.

Risk assessment is a major component of the patient's care plan and should be seen as an integral aspect of the overall medical and nursing assessment processes. The non-specialist's role is to assess risk in relation to the immediate nursing and medical management. Specialist mental health staff will undertake a more detailed or specific risk assessment, but the role of the general nurse is to undertake an initial assessment at the point of attendance or admission to hospital for the following reasons:

■ to clarify whether the person is at risk of further self-harm or suicide in the short term
■ to identify those risk factors that will inform the patient's immediate care and treatment
■ to ascertain whether the person is at long-term risk, so that specialist referral and follow up can be arranged if necessary.

It is important to consider how one will approach the assessment of risk, and this will be informed by:

■ the type of self-harming behaviour that the person presents with
■ the attitude and behaviour of the person on arrival or admission, for example, the degree of co-operativeness, level of consciousness, degree of intoxication
■ the information available from other sources, for example, written information brought in by the patient, information from partner, friends or significant others, and access to the person's medical and nursing history.

Information that will inform risk assessment can be obtained through observation, the use of questions and reference to sources of written information. There are no published examples of widely accepted and validated risk assessment tools designed specifically for use by non-mental health staff within this setting. Certain risk assessment tools do exist, but their applicability and reliability in such settings have not been tested. It is therefore necessary to consider such an assessment from a broader perspective, while attempting to identify those risk indicators that identify an increase in risk for the time that you are responsible for the person's care.

Certain groups of individuals have been identified as being at increased risk of suicide (Table 8.6), although it is important to remember that this information has been obtained after studying groups or populations, which limits its usefulness in the clinical situation and in particular when trying to make judgements concerning ongoing risk. For example, males are statistically at greater risk than females, yet knowing this when caring for a man who has harmed himself does not give us any information about his individual level of ongoing risk. However, the knowledge that males as a population are at increased risk of suicide is helpful in planning targeted suicide prevention strategies for high-risk groups (DoH, 2003b).

It is necessary to consider risk assessment in the context of the individual, their circumstances, the predisposing and precipitating factors to the act, their current thoughts and feelings, and whether there are any psychiatric symptoms present. Consideration needs to be given to the clinical features of the person's presentation and the identification of relevant risk characteristics from this aspect of the assessment (Hart *et al.*, 2005). A format for undertaking an initial assessment of risk is provided in Fig. 8.2.

Risk assessment is not a static concept, instead it is something that can fluctuate and vary over short periods of time. Various factors will influence the person's level of risk, and for this reason it is helpful to consider its assessment in relation to the short, medium and long term.

Short-term risk assessment

Is the person likely to act on thoughts of self-harm in the short term? Being aware of this will help in making decisions regarding the priority that needs to be attached to obtaining a specialist assessment, or the level of supervision or observation required while in the department or unit. This information is best obtained by direct questioning of the patient, encouraging them to be as specific as possible about the likelihood of acting on their suicidal thoughts.

Medium-term risk assessment

Some individuals retain suicidal thoughts, but deny any plans to act on them in the short term. However, they may be suffering from an ongoing mental

Table 8.6 Factors, situations and symptoms associated with increased risk of suicide and self-harm.

Individual
Single, divorced, widowed or separated
Access to potentially lethal means of harm/further harm, e.g. large amounts of
    medication, firearms
Physical illness – especially chronic, painful, debilitating and terminal conditions
Family history of suicide
Bereavement – especially loss of spouse/partner

Social
Living alone
Social isolation
Prisoners – especially those on remand

Psychiatric and psychological
Depression
Psychotic illness
Personality disorders
Substance misuse
History of self-harm

Clinical
Depressed thinking
Suicidal ideas
Suicidal plans
Expressions of hopelessness
Extreme variations in mood (lability) within relatively short periods of time –
    'mood swings'
Displays of hostility and aggression
Perceptual disturbance – particularly auditory hallucinations instructing the
    person to harm themselves

High-risk situations
Recent major stress, e.g. relationship breakdown, loss of employment
Recent self-harm
Currently receiving psychiatric inpatient care – especially if on 'leave'
    from hospital
Recent discharge from psychiatric inpatient care – especially during the first
    week following discharge
Anniversary of previously stressful or traumatic life event(s)
Ready access to potentially lethal means, e.g. farmers, vets

Indications of suicide risk following an episode of self-harm
Evidence of pre-planning
Well thought through and considered decision to choose a violent method
Fully expects or expected to die
Took steps to avoid discovery or intervention
Consciously isolated at the time of the act
Suicide note
Regret at survival

Assessment categories		
1. Background history and general observations	**Yes**	**No**
■ Does the person pose an immediate risk to self, you or others?		
■ Does the person have any *immediate* (i.e. within the next few minutes or hours) plans to harm self or others?		
■ Is the person aggressive and/or threatening?		
■ Is there any suggestion or does it appear likely that the person may try to abscond?		
■ Has the person got a history of self-harm?		
■ Does the person have a history of mental health problems or psychiatric illness?		
If yes to any of the above, record details below:		
2. Appearance and behaviour	**Yes**	**No**
■ Is the person obviously distressed, markedly anxious or highly aroused?		
■ Is the person behaving inappropriately to the situation?		
■ Is the person quiet and withdrawn?		
■ Is the person inattentive and unco-operative?		
If yes to any of the above, record details below:		
3. Issues to be explored through brief questioning		
■ Why is the person presenting now? What recent event(s) precipitated or triggered this presentation?		
■ What is the person's level of social support (i.e. partner/significant other, family members, friends)?		

4. Suicide risk screen – greater number of positive responses suggests greater level of overall risk

	yes	no	d/k		yes	no	d/k
Previous self-harm	☐	☐	☐	Family history of suicide	☐	☐	☐
Previous use of violent methods	☐	☐	☐	Unemployed/retired	☐	☐	☐
Suicide plan/expressed intent	☐	☐	☐	Male gender	☐	☐	☐
Current suicidal thoughts/ideation	☐	☐	☐	Separated/widowed/divorced	☐	☐	☐
Hopelessness/helplessness	☐	☐	☐	Lack of social support	☐	☐	☐
Depression	☐	☐	☐	Family concerned about risk	☐	☐	☐
Evidence of psychosis	☐	☐	☐	Disengaged from services	☐	☐	☐
Alcohol and/or drug misuse	☐	☐	☐	Poor adherence to psychiatric Tx	☐	☐	☐
Chronic physical illness/pain	☐	☐	☐	Access to lethal means of harm	☐	☐	☐

Action plan and outcomes following initial risk screen:
Describe all actions and interventions following assessment. Include details of referral to other team(s), telephone calls/advice and discharge/transfer or follow-up plans.

Figure 8.2 Overview of the risk assessment process.

illness or another psychological problem that requires specialist assessment or treatment. Some individuals may describe ongoing suicidal thoughts, but despite this may have no plans to act on them in the short term. For a number of patients, self-harm may be the culmination of a long period of distressing symptoms and difficulties. In order to manage and reduce the associated risks, it is important to ensure that such patients are referred on for appropriate specialist help.

Long-term risk assessment

Statistically, all individuals who have self-harmed have an increased risk of suicide in the long term. For a number of patients the act of self-harm was 'a one-off', an out-of-character action that they find difficult to explain and does not reflect how he or she is currently thinking and feeling. However, a number of these individuals may have long-standing difficulties with communication, or in maintaining effective interpersonal relationships, that predispose them to the risk of further self-harm or suicide in the long term.

Caring for the person who has self-harmed

The nursing aims when caring for a person who has engaged in self-harm are:

■ to assess and treat the physical complications of the self-harming behaviour in order to prevent or minimise the risk of disability or death
■ to undertake an initial assessment of risk
■ to ensure that the patient receives the most appropriate treatment, help and support for any underlying mental health or psychological problems.

A comprehensive care plan will ensure that the patient is cared for in an atmosphere of respect and understanding. It is important to remember that, like many patients, the person who has self-harmed is likely to feel confused, anxious and low in mood. Therefore, nursing interventions should aim to provide reassurance, explanation and psychological support.

Initial assessment

Initial assessment of risk is a priority and specific areas to be addressed are identified in Fig. 8.2. The key nursing responsibilities during this phase are:

Risk assessment
Ensure that an initial risk assessment has been undertaken, and explain to the patient why you need to ask questions about this. Ask specific questions pertaining to the person's attitude and thoughts about further self-harm or suicide (Box 8.3). It is important not to avoid direct questions concerning the person's thoughts or plans regarding further self-harm, as in this way risk

---

Box 8.3 Questioning techniques following self-harm.

'What things have led up to you harming yourself?'
'What did you want to, or what did you think would, happen as a result of you harming yourself?'
'Do you still have any thoughts or plans to harm yourself?'
'How likely do you think you are to act on these thoughts?' It is often helpful to suggest that the person uses a 0–10 analogue scale to rate the likelihood of further self-harm, i.e. 0 = will definitely not harm myself, 10 = will definitely harm myself
'How do you feel now about having harmed yourself?'
'Do you have anything on you now that you could harm yourself with while you are in hospital?'

---

can be assessed and managed more effectively, and the person may experience relief that previously distressing feelings can now be discussed openly and honestly. The risk assessment format identified in Fig. 8.2 should be followed.

Effective interpersonal communication

Many patients will feel ashamed, guilty and embarrassed at having self-harmed, and one of the most important needs is for the staff caring for them to understand this distress and to provide a degree of psychological support (Hart, 2003). In order to ensure that the person feels supported and understood, a number of key factors underpin the nurse's approach to care (Box 8.4).

Box 8.4 Critical factors relating to effective interpersonal communication.

Adopt a non-judgemental and non-critical attitude. Overt or implied criticism only serves to reinforce the person's sense of guilt and shame
Observe and note details of the person's behaviour, in particular whether he or she is angry, impulsive, irritable, withdrawn or tearful
Use the skills of active listening. This will assist in engaging the person in the processes of assessment and care
Use open questions as a means of gaining a more detailed understanding of the person's emotional state, such as, 'How are you feeling now?', 'What would help you deal with your current difficulties?'
Acknowledge the person's underlying distress by using empathic responses such as, 'I can see you are very upset', 'You look distressed', 'You must have found it very hard coping with these feelings of depression'
Avoid the use of overly reassuring statements, such as promising things that it may be difficult to deliver, such as, 'Everything will be all right', 'Don't worry, we'll sort all your problems out'

Treatment

The patient will require specific care relating to the treatment of their physical injury or complications as a result of the self-harm. All patients who attend or are admitted following self-harm should be closely observed for any deterioration in their physical state, psychological distress and any additional self-harming behaviour. The development of care planning guidance for staff is a useful way of assisting with the provision of care for this group of patients (Kadum, 2001; Littlejohn, 2004).

Managing the potential risk of further self-harm

A small number of individuals may retain suicidal thoughts and plans to such an extent that they continue to actively contemplate further self-harm while in hospital. If the patient describes such thoughts, it is important to clarify how likely they are to act on them. In particular, a direct question regarding whether they have any means of harming themselves, such as medication or sharp objects, should be asked. If this is the case, the person should be asked to hand these over for safe keeping while in hospital.

Observation

The person should be nursed in an area that allows easy observation and regular eye contact by staff. However, a balance must be struck between ensuring that staff know the patient's whereabouts and their need for privacy. If specific risks of repetition or suicide have been identified, then a further assessment and advice from specialist mental health staff should be sought.

Pre-discharge care

Planning for discharge is one of the most important aspects of the person's care. For many individuals, the act of self-harm may be a means of communicating distress relating to underlying interpersonal, family or social difficulties. It would not be realistic to expect to deal with all such difficulties while the person is in hospital, but these may require referral, advice and specialist assessment by other members of the health care team.

If the person absconds or disappears from hospital before a discharge plan has been agreed, or before a specialist psychosocial assessment has taken place, the nurse will need to consider what actions to take in order to ensure that follow-up care can be arranged. Such actions will also demonstrate how the nurse and the organisation will address the duty of care they owe the patient. Deciding what actions are appropriate in such a situation will be informed by the baseline risk assessment undertaken on arrival or admission to hospital (Box 8.5).

> **Box 8.5** Nursing actions should a person leave hospital before discharge plans have been agreed.
>
> Refer to information contained in baseline risk assessment
> Follow your organisation's 'Missing Patient/Person Policy'
> Inform nearest relative or significant other/family member
> Inform patient's general practitioner (GP) and other professional carers (e.g. community psychiatric nurse (CPN)), if appropriate
> If baseline assessment has identified significant short-term suicide risk, seek advice from senior colleague about whether there is a need to inform the police of the fact that the patient is missing

> **Box 8.6** Information required before discharging a patient who has self-harmed.
>
> All relevant documentation completed, e.g. risk assessment
> Patient has been assessed as medically and physically well enough to leave hospital
> Referral organised to mental health staff for psychosocial assessment
> Relative/significant other informed of discharge plans
> Written information and advice provided
> Patient's GP informed
> If person is already known to secondary mental health services, the person's key worker or care co-ordinator informed
> If decision to discharge patient without psychosocial assessment, reasons for this fully documented

All individuals who have self-harmed should be offered a specialist psychosocial assessment by a mental health professional. On occasions, it may not be possible or appropriate to arrange this before the person leaves hospital. If this is the case, the patient should be made aware of how to access further help and support once they return home. A list of key nursing tasks prior to discharge home is provided in Box 8.6.

Conclusions

Self-harm is a common reason why individuals attend hospital, yet many staff struggle to maintain a positive approach to the assessment and care for this group of patients. In order to develop the professional confidence and skills in this area it is necessary for nurses to understand the reasons why people engage in self-harming behaviour, as well as the core principles involved in assessing need and planning care. With such high rates of self-harming behaviour, it is important for all practitioners working in non-mental health settings to develop these skills.

This chapter has provided an overview of the main reasons why people may engage in self-harm, alongside a discussion of the impact that staff attitudes may have upon the individual. It suggests that non-mental health staff have a key role to play in the assessment of risk and in ensuring that those patients who require ongoing specialist help are identified following attendance at hospital. Undertaking such a role is one means by which general hospital staff can contribute to reducing suicide rates, positively promote mental health, reduce stigma and improve access to treatment for people with a range of psychological and mental health problems.

References

Babiker, B. & Arnold, L. (1997) *The Language of Injury: comprehending self-mutilation.* Leicester: British Psychological Society.

Brinn, F. (2000) Patients with mental illness: general nurses' attitudes and expectations. *Nursing Standard*, 14 (27): 32–36.

Department of Health (2003a) *Essence of Care: patient focused benchmarks for clinical governance.* London: DoH.

Department of Health (2003b) *National Suicide Prevention Strategy for England: annual report on progress 2003.* London: DoH.

Department of Health and Social Security (1984) *The Management of Deliberate Self-Harm.* London: DHSS.

Gairin, I., House, A. & Owens, D. (2003) Attendance at the accident and emergency department in the year before suicide: a retrospective study. *British Journal of Psychiatry*, 183: 28–33.

Gelder, M., Mayou, R. & Geddes, J. (1999) *Psychiatry*, 2nd edn. Oxford: Oxford University Press.

Greenwood, S. & Bradley, P. (1997) Managing deliberate self-harm: the A&E perspective. *Accident and Emergency Nursing*, 5: 134–136.

Harris, F.C. & Barraclough, B.M. (1994) Suicide as an outcome for medical disorders. *Medicine*, 73 (6): 281–298.

Hart, C., Colley, R. & Harrison, A. (2005) Using a risk assessment matrix with mental health patients in emergency departments. *Emergency Nurse*, 12 (9): 21–28.

Hart, L. (2003) Are you suicidal? *Openmind* 120, March/April: 8.

Hawton, K. & Fagg, J. (1992) Trends in deliberate self-poisoning and self-injury in Oxford 1976–90. *British Medical Journal*, 317: 441–447.

Hawton, K., Fagg, J. & Simkin, S. (1997) Trends in deliberate self-poisoning in Oxford, 1985–1995: Implications for clinical services and the prevention of suicide. *British Journal of Psychiatry*, 171, 556–560.

Hawton, K. & van Heeringen, K. (2000) *The International Handbook of Suicide and Attempted Suicide.* Chichester: John Wiley & Sons.

Hawton, K., Ware, C. & Kingsbury, S. (1996) Paracetamol self-poisoning: characteristics, prevention and harm reduction. *British Journal of Psychiatry*, 168 (1): 43–48.

Hemmings, A. (1999) Attitudes to deliberate self-harm among staff in an accident and emergency team. *Mental Health Care*, 2 (9): 300–302.

Hopkins, C. (2002) 'But what about the really ill, poorly people?' *Journal of Psychiatric and Mental Health Nursing*, 9: 147–154.

Horrocks, J., Price, S. & House, A. (2003) Self-injury attendances in the accident and emergency department. *British Journal of Psychiatry*, 183: 34–39.

Hunt, E. (1993) On avoiding 'psych' patients. *Journal of Emergency Nursing*, 19 (5): 375–376.

James, R. (2004) Cut it out, please. *Guardian*, 3 August: 16.

Kadum, D. (2001) NT Practice solutions. *Nursing Times*, 97 (30): 44.

Kerkhof, A.J.F.M. (2000) Attempted suicide: patterns and trends. In: K. Hawton & K. van Heeringen (eds) *The International Handbook of Suicide and Attempted Suicide*, pp. 49–64. Chichester: John Wiley & Sons.

Littlejohn, C. (2004) Understanding the nurse's role in improving suicide prevention. *Nursing Times*, 100 (46): 28–29.

Lynn, F. (1998) The pain of rejection. *Nursing Times*, 94 (27): 36.

Murray, I. (1998) At the cutting edge. *Nursing Times*, 94 (27): 36–37.

National Institute for Clinical Excellence (2004) *Self-harm: the short-term physical and psychological management and secondary prevention of self-harm in primary and secondary care*. Clinical Guideline 16. London: NICE.

Pembroke, L. (2000) Damage limitation. *Nursing Times*, 96 (34): 34–35.

Perego, M. (1999) Why A&E nurses feel inadequate in managing patients who deliberately self-harm. *Emergency Nurse*, 6 (9): 24–27.

Richardson, C. (2004) Self-harm: understanding the causes and treatment options. *Nursing Times*, 100 (15): 24–25.

Roberts, D. (1996) Suicide prevention by general nurses. *Nursing Standard*, 10 (17): 30–33.

Stenager, E.N. & Stenager, E. (2000) Physical illness and suicidal behaviour. In: K. Hawton & K. van Heeringen (eds) *The International Handbook of Suicide and Attempted Suicide*, pp. 405–420. Chichester: John Wiley & Sons.

Chapter 9
Perinatal and Maternal Mental Health

Chapter aims

This chapter will:

- identify the common mental health problems that occur during the perinatal period
- describe the relevant vulnerability factors and risk characteristics associated with the development of perinatal mental health problems
- describe the assessment, treatment and clinical management of perinatal depression and puerperal psychosis
- identify the proactive role of midwives and health visitors in the screening, assessment and care of women experiencing mental health problems during the perinatal period.

Introduction

Childbirth and pregnancy are significant and complex events accompanied by numerous physical and psychological responses. They are periods of rapid biological, social and emotional transition, which permanently change the status and responsibilities of a woman's life (Brockington, 1996). For most women giving birth is a positive event that is unequalled, however, for some, pregnancy and childbirth can be traumatic experiences that precipitate significant mental health difficulties. The perinatal period is generally considered to cover the time from conception to 12 months following childbirth.

Failing to address perinatal mental health issues can lead to multiple health and social problems. The potential consequences of untreated mental health difficulties may include poor maternal and infant health, increased maternal and infant morbidity, child development delays and behavioural problems, parental relationship difficulties, and even suicide and infanticide.

Policy and professional context

Recent health policy in the United Kingdom has recognised perinatal mental health as an area that needs attention from all those who have responsibility to provide health services for pregnant women and new mothers. The *National Service Framework for Mental Health* (Department of Health (DoH), 1999) highlights the incidence of mental illness in the postnatal period and emphasises the increased risk of suicide among mothers following childbirth. It requires organisations to develop protocols which address early detection and management of such problems in primary care, through to specialist treatments in maternity units and secondary care services. In order to ensure integrated care from early pregnancy through to the postpartum period, a number of recommendations have been made that focus on early detection and prompt intervention, alongside co-ordinated and collaborative care (DoH, 2003).

Despite the identified need and drive to improve mental health care, perinatal provision is generally patchy and there is evidence that the lack of co-ordinated and specialist services during this period can lead to fatally tragic consequences (Confidential Enquiry into Maternal Deaths, 2001; Confidential Enquiries into Maternal and Child Health, 2004). An issue of importance for midwives, health visitors and nurses is the erroneous view that the perinatal period is the exclusive domain of one professional group, leading to 'tribal' attitudes and a lack of collaborative and co-ordinated professional practice (Currid, 2004). In reality, all health care professionals have a potential role to play in ensuring that perinatal care is delivered in the most appropriate and timely manner.

An enhanced public health role has been identified for nurses, midwives and health visitors in the provision of perinatal health care (DoH, 1999, 2004). One area for development involves the early detection and screening of people with mental health problems. Included in this is the need to develop roles that promote health in communities as well as in individuals, by acting as advocates for people to ensure that they access health care in a timely and appropriate way. This agenda specifically challenges health care staff to provide enhanced services for individuals who are vulnerable at critical stages of the life cycle, such as during pregnancy and following childbirth.

Health visitors and midwives are in the unique position of being in contact with people when they are well. Women's contact with the health service is greater during pregnancy than at any other time and should in theory present an ideal opportunity to meet their psychological needs (Clark, 2000; Price, 2004). In addition, the woman will see her general practitioner (GP) regularly and may also be seen by fertility experts, gynaecology staff and an obstetric team. The scope for mental health promotion, health education, symptom detection, illness prevention and treatment during this period should be utilised to the full.

Regardless of national or local models of care provision, midwives and health visitors maintain a pivotal role in supporting mothers and families during this time. A number of organisations have taken a proactive approach and have developed services that have responded to this public health agenda and service gap. Examples such as those linked to Sure Start Programmes and inter-service 'fast track' referral systems demonstrate the development of innovative and creative approaches to meeting perinatal mental health need (Davies *et al.*, 2003).

Prevalence of perinatal mental health problems

Perinatal mental health problems can present in a number of ways and range in significance from those that are mild and transitory to those that may be accompanied by a range of severe and distressing symptoms (Box 9.1).

There is evidence of the health consequences for the family, with fathers experiencing an increase in mental health problems, as well as an increased risk of general health problems (Harvey & McGrath, 1988). The babies of mothers with mental health problems have an increased risk of developing problems in their own right, including attachment insecurity, emotional development delay and poor social interactions with other children (Murray *et al.*, 1999). Of particular note are the effects that postnatal depression can have on baby boys, who have been found to have insecure attachments at 18 months and a high level of frank behavioural disturbance at the age of 5 years (Cooper & Murray, 1998).

The prevalence of postnatal depression is approximately 10%. In women with a history of mental illness, two in every 1000 will require inpatient admission as a result of an exacerbation of their psychiatric illness (Royal College of Psychiatrists, 2000). Those women who have a history of a psychotic mental illness have a higher incidence of stillbirth and neonatal death (Howard *et al.*, 2004). The development of perinatal mental health problems may be associated with, or aggravated by, a number of factors including:

- Psychological – social and personal expectations of being a mother, psychological effects of a traumatic delivery.
- Social – social isolation, economic status, ethnicity, cultural issues and accommodation and housing difficulties.
- Family – relationship with the child's father, level of support and help received from family and friends.
- Biological – genetic predisposition, hormonal changes that occur during pregnancy, childbirth and postpartum.
- Personal – alcohol use, illicit and prescribed drug use, domestic/relationship violence, childhood sexual abuse, previous history of mental health problems, maternal history.
- The infant's general health.

> **Box 9.1** Most common perinatal mental health problems (Brockington, 2004).
>
> ■ Postpartum psychoses
> ■ Disorders affecting the mother–infant relationship
> ■ Depression
> ■ Post-traumatic stress disorder (PTSD)
> ■ Morbid preoccupations
> ■ Anxiety specific to the puerperium
> ■ Obsessions of child harm

The impact of mental illness

Women are vulnerable during pregnancy and the postpartum period to developing mental health problems and to experiencing a relapse of an existing mental illness (Royal College of Psychiatrists, 2000). The needs of women with pre-existing mental illnesses are often overlooked and assumptions are made regarding the involvement of services. Some women are reluctant to disclose their involvement with mental health services and this is thought to be one of the factors related to the relatively high levels of custody loss in women who have an existing psychiatric illness (Howard, 2000). Approximately 12% of maternal deaths are linked to psychiatric illness, with suicide being a major reason for mortality in this group (Confidential Enquiry into Maternal Deaths, 2001). Any psychological or mental health problem experienced by the mother has the potential to cause long-term detrimental effects on the child's and family's adjustment, communication and psychological functioning (Cooper & Murray, 1998).

Those women who are depressed during pregnancy are more likely to continue feeling depressed during the postnatal period (Evans *et al.*, 2001). Some may have an abnormal fear of pregnancy, feeling extremely anxious and distressed; such a fear is known as tokophobia. Women who experience postnatal depression describe feeling robbed of what should have been a happy time in their lives (Cox *et al.*, 1993). Stein *et al.* (1991) found a link between postnatal depression and negative mother–child interaction and bonding. In general, those women who experienced depression were less facilitating as mothers, and their children demonstrated less emotional sharing and sociability with strangers at 2 and 3 years old.

Common perinatal mental health problems

There are a number of common mental health problems associated with the perinatal period and a number of risk factors have been identified in their development (Box 9.2).

> **Box 9.2** Risk factors for the development of perinatal mental health problems.
>
> - Social factors, e.g. poverty, housing and accommodation problems, lack of social support and confiding personal networks
> - Poor interpersonal/marital relationship
> - Recent adverse life events, e.g. bereavement, unemployment, etc.
> - Psychological problems and difficulties during pregnancy
> - History of mental illness
> - 'Maternity blues'
> - Neonatal factors, e.g. infant irritability, poor motor control, etc.

Maternity or baby blues

This is a transient mood change occurring about four days postpartum, when the mother may become tearful. It is a mild and self-limiting condition, usually characterised by labile mood, tearfulness, anxiety, irritability, headaches and mild forgetfulness (Brockington, 1996). The woman may appear up and down in mood, happy one minute and weeping the next, and may be viewed as being over sensitive to comments. The 'blues' last for two or three days and may peak on day five. Although there is no specific treatment, it is important to have an understanding of the condition, as it is often a distressing and perplexing period for the mother and family. It responds well to explanation, emotional support and reassurance.

Postnatal depression

Depression can affect every aspect of an individual's feelings, thoughts and functions and is commonly associated with a range of physical health problems and illnesses. Postnatal depression is important because of its incidence and in view of the fact that it occurs at such a significant period in the lives of the mother, her baby and the family. It affects between 10% and 15% of women, although the onset is variable and can occur at any time during the first year postpartum, the peak time for occurrence is at five weeks (Cox *et al.*, 1993).

Depression after childbirth is clinically similar to other depressive disorders and the consensus view is that its cause is multi-factorial, although there is no clear evidence as to a specific hormonal or biological basis (Lee *et al.*, 2000) (see Chapter 7). Green (1998) challenges the speed with which depression is diagnosed postnatally, pointing out that any new mother can reasonably expect to experience a range of emotions following childbirth, yet these may not in themselves constitute an episode of clinical depression. Green also argues that similar numbers of women are depressed in the antenatal period as those who are depressed following delivery. Evans *et al.* (2001) suggest that there is as much (or more) depression antenatally as postnatally, so there should be more focus on diagnosing and treating antenatal depression rather than the almost exclusive concentration on postnatal depression.

The term postnatal depression is used to describe a persistent depressive disorder in women following childbirth and is characterised by:

- Low, sad mood
- Loss of interest in oneself, the infant and family life
- Lack of interest
- Increased anxiety
- Disturbed sleep
- Somatic (physical) symptoms
- Reduced motivation and difficulty completing day-to-day tasks.

Identifying and confirming depression during this period can be problematic, in particular due to the fact that the experience of childbirth is new and often unfamiliar. If depression is suspected, a clinical assessment is required in order to understand and contextualise the experience for the mother and family. Table 9.1 provides an overview of the signs and symptoms of postnatal depression, although many of these symptoms will be present in both antenatal and postnatal depression.

The detection and identification of postnatal depression is a priority for all staff, in particular midwives and health visitors. Both play a potentially vital role in identifying women at highest risk. Mothers undergo a six-week postnatal examination and babies undergo a routine post-delivery health check at eight weeks, making these ideal opportunities to undertake formal screening for mental health problems. Various screening tools exist to assist in the detection of depression in vulnerable groups (see Chapter 7), and depression screening has been advocated as a key aspect of postnatal care by health visitors (Davies *et al.*, 2003). A number of screening tools have been developed, including:

- Edinburgh Postnatal Depression Scale (EPDS) (Cox *et al.*, 1987)
- Postpartum Depression Screening Scale (Beck, 2003)

The EPDS (Box 9.3) is a self-report scale devised as a screening questionnaire that seeks to detect postnatal depression and can be completed in approximately ten minutes. It can be administered by any health professional for use with women in the postnatal period, and its use is now advocated as part of routine mother and child health checks (Bewley, 2000). It has been shown to be effective in identifying those women at high risk and increased likelihood of experiencing postnatal depression (Cox *et al.*, 1993).

The EPDS was developed as a simple means of screening for postnatal depression in health care settings. It contains ten statements each with four responses, and the woman is asked to underline one response that comes closest to how she has felt during the preceding seven days. A cut-off score

Table 9.1 Overview of the signs and symptoms of postnatal depression.

Psychological	
Persistent low mood	Crying and tearfulness Intense tearfulness and mood swings, often triggered by insignificant remarks or comments from others Intense feelings of sadness Difficulty in demonstrating love and overt affection for the infant
Anhedonia	Loss of pleasure, in particular, no pleasure from new maternal role No interest in infant's developmental milestones Failure or difficulty in responding to comments and feedback from others, such as family members Leaving others (e.g. partner, grandparents, older children) to take the lead with the infant Loss of libido
Feelings of guilt	Feelings of not being a good enough mother or of being inadequate in new role Irrational self-blame and criticism for minor infant complaints, such as nappy rash, colic, teething, etc.
Low self-esteem	Feelings of hopelessness, worthlessness and helplessness, and feeling a failure
Anxiety over the infant's health	Preoccupation with the baby's health, such as minor feeding problems, sleep pattern, crying, etc.
Impaired concentration	Difficulty remembering time of last feed or nappy change Unable to concentrate on reading, watching TV, etc.
Impaired mother–infant interaction	Little interaction with baby Limited face to face gazing Appearing emotionally detached and disconnected from the infant
Biological	
Physical	May experience early morning awakening when not disturbed by baby Difficulty returning to sleep following night feeds Appetite loss Non-specific somatic complaints – aches, abdominal and breast pains, feelings of lethargy
Lethargy	Tired all the time, unable to complete daily tasks, e.g. laundry, meal preparation Remaining in night clothes during the daytime Personal neglect Physical care of the baby adversely affected

Box 9.3 The Edinburgh Postnatal Depression Scale.

Question

In the past 7 days:

(1) I have been able to laugh and see the funny side of things:
- As much as I always could
- Not quite so much now
- Definitely not so much now
- Not at all

(2) I have looked forward with enjoyment to things:
- As much as I ever did
- Rather less than I used to
- Definitely less than I used to
- Hardly at all

(3) I have blamed myself unnecessarily when things went wrong:
- Yes, most of the time
- Yes, some of the time
- Not very often
- No, never

(4) I have been anxious or worried for no good reason:
- No, not at all
- Hardly ever
- Yes, sometimes
- Yes, very often

(5) I have felt scared or panicky for no good reason:
- Yes, quite a lot
- Yes, sometimes
- No, not much
- No, not at all

(6) Things have been getting on top of me:
- Yes, most of the time I haven't been able to cope at all
- Yes, sometimes I haven't been coping as well as usual
- No, most of the time I have coped quite well
- No, I have been coping as well as ever

(7) I have been so unhappy that I have had difficulty sleeping:
- Yes, most of the time
- Yes, sometimes
- Not very often
- No, not at all

(8) I have felt sad or miserable:
- Yes, most of the time
- Yes, quite often
- Not very often
- No, not at all

Box 9.3 (*Cont'd*)

(9) I have been so unhappy that I have been crying:
- Yes, most of the time
- Yes, quite often
- Only occasionally
- No, never

(10) The thought of harming myself has occurred to me:
- Yes, quite often
- Sometimes
- Hardly ever
- Never

Response categories are scored 0, 1, 2 and 3, according to increased severity of the symptom.

Questions 3, 5, 6, 7, 8, 9, 10 are reverse scored (i.e. response categories are scored 3, 2, 1, and 0 according to increased severity of the symptom)

Individual items are totalled to give an overall score. A score of 12+ indicates the likelihood of depression, but not its severity.

© 1987 The Royal College of Psychiatrists. The Edinburgh Postnatal Depression Scale may be photocopied by individual researchers or clinicians for their own use without seeking permission from the publishers. The scale must be copied in full and all copies must acknowledge the following source: Cox, J.L., Holden, J.M. & Sagovsky, R. (1987) Detection of postnatal depression. Development of the 10-item Edinburgh Postnatal Depression Scale. *British Journal of Psychiatry*, **150**, 782–786. Written permission must be obtained from the Royal College of Psychiatrists for copying and distribution to others or for republication (in print, online or by any other medium). Translations of the scale, and guidance to its use, may be found in Cox, J.L. & Holden, J. (2003) *Perinatal Mental Health: A Guide to the Edinburgh Postnatal Depression Scale*. London: Gaskell.

of >12 is used to identify those women who are more likely to be depressed, although it has been advocated that a lower score of >10 is likely to reduce the number of false negative scores and improve the identification of those women who are depressed (Buist *et al.*, 2002). As with all other screening tools it should not be used in isolation, or form the only source of information regarding the woman's mental state, but should be part of an holistic post-partum assessment. It is not a diagnostic tool, and positive scoring should be followed up with a more detailed clinical assessment to clarify the symptoms and identify any co-existing morbidity (Brockington, 2004).

Postnatal depression is a highly treatable condition; however, the symptoms are commonly missed (Cooper & Murray, 1998). Buist *et al.* (2002) recognise the difficulties inherent in screening for both antenatal and postnatal depression, in particular the lack of consensus regarding the most appropriate screening tools to use. However, on balance the advantages of screening for depression during this time outweigh the disadvantages and problems associated with the process (Buist *et al.*, 2002), and midwives have clear guidance that the EPDS should not be used routinely during the antenatal period (National Collaborating Centre for Women's and Children's Health, 2003). Treatment measures include antidepressants and non-directive counselling or interpersonal psychotherapy (see Chapter 7). The principal challenge remains the more effective screening, risk assessment and identification of the illness (Hendrick, 2003).

Puerperal psychosis

For every 1000 live births, between one and two (0.2%) mothers will develop a puerperal psychosis (Oates, 1996). Puerperal psychosis is an acute and severe mental illness, with a typically sudden and rapid onset. It usually develops during the ten days following delivery, but may also occur within a few hours. There is no conclusive evidence as to specific differences between psychosis following childbirth and other forms of psychotic illness experienced at other periods of life. Symptoms are consistent with those observed in other forms of severe mental illness, such as schizophrenia, bipolar affective disorder and severe depression (see Chapter 10). However, despite the debate regarding the concept of puerperal psychosis, it is important for practitioners to be aware of the possibility of such a presentation and deliver care that is person-focused and needs-led; it is the mother's needs that arise as a result of such a presentation that are central to the care planning process, as opposed to any arbitrary classification of the illness itself (Currid, 2004).

Although puerperal psychosis is rare, its symptoms are serious and its severe and disabling nature can have a profound effect on a woman at a fundamental period in her life. Identifying those at risk is not easy or straightforward, although the following factors are likely to reflect an increase in overall risk of developing the syndrome (Kendell *et al.*, 1987):

- Past history of puerperal psychosis
- First time mother
- Caesarean section
- Perinatal infant death
- Pre-existing psychotic illness
- Family history of mood disorder.

The illness is characterised by a dramatic change in mental state and a pronounced disturbance of mood, which can be consistently low or high, or fluctuate unpredictably between the two extremes (DoH, 2003). The onset is typically acute – after a lucid, and apparently 'normal' period, the mother's mental state can dramatically change and she displays florid symptoms across a spectrum of acute mental illness (Table 9.2). The symptoms are typically those of mania, depression and psychosis.

Although the incidence is low, the severity of the condition can mean that the mother deteriorates rapidly and dangerously. There is limited evidence

Table 9.2 Common features of puerperal psychosis (Gaskell, 1999).

Predisposition and background factors	Severe, but relatively uncommon form of postnatal mental illness Rapid onset – symptoms typically presenting 48–72 hours postpartum or within two weeks of delivery Occurs across ethnic groups, countries and cultures Occurs most frequently after the first delivery
Depressive features	Depressed mood Frequent crying Suicidal thoughts Significantly impaired concentration Stupor Somatic symptoms including loss of appetite, markedly disturbed sleep pattern
Features of an elevated mood (mania or hypomania)	Elated mood which may fluctuate rapidly Unrealistic feelings of wellbeing Marked over-activity Restlessness and agitation Little need for sleep or rest
Psychotic features	Delusions – often related to the baby Hallucinations Intrusive thoughts Unusual beliefs Confusion or perplexity

regarding preventative interventions during pregnancy, although the use of prophylactic mood stabilisers such as lithium postpartum has demonstrated effectiveness in the prevention of a subsequent episode (Cohen *et al.*, 1995).

The role of the midwife, health visitor and nurse centres on the immediate assessment, sensitive clinical management and skilled physical and psychological care of the mother, plus protection and safety of the baby. This will include an immediate referral to, and effective liaison with, mental health professionals for assessment and treatment. The safety needs of the baby are paramount and in certain circumstances the child may need to be temporarily removed from the mother. This may include the infant being cared for within an alternative part of the clinical unit, or its needs may best be met by temporary responsibility for its care passing to a close relative or guardian, such as the father or grandparents. Staff should follow locally agreed child protection guidelines and seek advice and supervision from senior colleagues as appropriate.

An important role for all health care staff focuses on secondary and tertiary prevention. Secondary prevention requires midwives and health visitors to maintain an awareness of the symptoms and features of puerperal psychosis, thereby ensuring speedy referral and access to mental health interventions.

Staff should be familiar with local guidelines and referral protocols, which should include a named professional contact in the mental health services who can facilitate an urgent assessment and provide advice and guidance for ongoing care and treatment (Royal College of Psychiatrists, 2000). Given that those mothers with the highest risk of developing puerperal psychosis are those with a pre-existing mental illness, good postpartum care is more likely to occur if there has been effective liaison and collaboration between mental health and obstetric services during the antenatal period.

The severity and acuteness of this illness requires urgent assessment and specialist treatment and often results in admission to a mental health unit. The midwife or health visitor should mobilise family help if available, including making arrangements for the immediate care of the baby. Any admission to hospital should ideally be of the woman and infant together to a specialised mother and baby unit (DoH, 1999). Local treatment will allow continued care from the midwife and health visitor.

Secondary prevention is paramount for women who have previously experienced an episode of puerperal psychosis (Box 9.4). From the first or second trimester there must be collaboration between maternity and mental health services for this small group of women. Although this may appear logical,

---

Box 9.4 Examples of secondary prevention activity for midwives and health visitors.

- Maintain up-to-date knowledge of symptoms and features of perinatal mental health issues and puerperal psychosis
- Identify women with a history of mental illness. At antenatal booking the midwife should ask whether there is any previous psychiatric history. If this is positive, then there is a need to sensitively explore and record:

  - care received, i.e. where, when, clinical team involved, admissions to hospital, follow up
  - clinical presentation, what form did the illness take?
  - severity – explore the woman's experience, e.g. was the baby at risk, subject to child protection procedures, was there any self-harming or suicidal behaviour?

- Be aware of local protocols and clinical guidelines, e.g. child protection procedures, contact details for local mental health services, etc.
- Involve partner and family – are they aware of the risk of recurrence, knowledge of clinical features, how will they access help should relapse occur?
- Collaborate with mental health services and the primary care team at early stage in antenatal period
- Ensure labour ward staff and obstetric team are aware of the potential for recurrence when the woman is admitted to hospital, and that a clinical management plan is available to midwifery staff

evidence demonstrates that this may not be consistent practice (Confidential Enquiries into Maternal and Child Health, 2004). All midwifes and health visitors need to be aware of the high risk of relapse in this group of individuals and, in order to respond appropriately, local protocols should encourage direct contact and referral between midwife and health visitor to mental health staff, including psychiatrists.

All mothers with a previous history of serious mental illness should be referred to the relevant mental health team to receive assessment by a psychiatrist in the antenatal period and a management plan should be instituted following childbirth (Confidential Enquiry into Maternal Deaths, 2001). If specialist input from mental health services is required, it is important that the mid-wife or health visitor remain involved during this period in order to ensure adequate attention is given to those aspects of care normally the responsibility of these staff. Active involvement from perinatal staff is of vital importance in ensuring continuity of care, effective communication and interprofessional working.

Treatment for puerperal psychosis will depend upon the exact nature of the clinical symptoms and will be consistent with treatment for the disorders as described in Chapter 10. Antipsychotics, antidepressants and mood stabilising medication may all be prescribed.

Breast feeding and the use of psychotropic medication

Breast milk offers a number of advantages to developing infants, and the process of breast feeding serves a number of important physical, psychological and practical advantages for both the mother and the baby (Nicholl & Williams, 2002). Breast feeding confers a number of benefits for the mother and infant, including lower rates of gastrointestinal disease, anaemia and respiratory problems, as well as providing a unique opportunity for bonding between the mother and child (Burt et al., 2001). Given the increased vulnerability to mental health problems during the postpartum period, women and their health professionals may face difficulty in deciding whether to commence treatment with psychotropic medication. The decision regarding whether to continue breast feeding when taking medication will be a complex one, influenced by a number of important factors (Box 9.5), and it is one that will require the midwife and health visitor to provide the mother and her family with additional support in order to reach it. Achieving concordance regarding the use of antidepressant medication in new mothers who are depressed is often difficult, and is likely to be even more so if the woman is breast feeding (Boath et al., 2004).

All psychotropic medication enters breast milk (Burt et al., 2001), although the effects of individual medications will vary between drug and individual mother. The amount of active psychotropic substance that is excreted is difficult to specify, and it is recommended that enhanced levels of observation of both the mother and the infant are undertaken when a woman who is taking

> **Box 9.5** Factors influencing the decision to prescribe medication in new mothers
>
> - Health benefits of breast feeding for the mother and infant
> - Mother's attitude and pre-existing views on mental illness, medication and breast feeding
> - Nature and symptoms of the mother's mental health difficulty
> - Degree of practical and emotional support available
> - Analysis of the potential risks of the excretion of medication (and its active metabolites) in breast milk and its possible effect on the infant
> - Attitude and advice of partner, family members and health professionals
> - Potential impact of untreated maternal mental illness on infant attachment and cognitive and behavioural development

psychotropic medication continues to breast feed. Limited data are available regarding the short- and long-term effects of the use of individual psychotropic agents on breast-feeding mothers and infants, although a number of antidepressant and antipsychotic medications have been used by breast-feeding mothers with no reported long-term risks to the infant (Spigset & Mårtensson, 1999; Burt *et al.*, 2001; Hendrick, 2003). However, the capacity for drug elimination in infants is significantly different from that of older children and adults, so even apparently insignificant amounts of the drug in breast milk may lead to problems (Spigset & Hägg, 1998). If it is necessary for medication to be taken by the mother, it should be administered immediately after breast feeding in order to limit the amount present in the milk and maximise metabolic clearance before the infant's next feed (Kacew, 1993).

Principles of effective perinatal mental health care

Effective perinatal mental health care is dependent upon:

- Collaboration and interdisciplinary working between and within health care teams, in particular effective liaison and joint working between primary health care, secondary mental health and maternity services. Such cross boundary working needs to be underpinned by appropriate policy and practice guidelines.
- Maternity and primary care staff who maintain an up-to-date knowledge and skills base regarding perinatal mental health issues, treatment and care.
- Development of specialist roles within primary care and maternity teams that focus on mental health care.
- Willingness by staff to challenge and stretch the boundaries of current professional practice, with the aim of delivering user-led care that meets the needs of women, children and families.

Box 9.6 Objectives of perinatal mental health care.

Maintenance of a safe environment for the mother and infant. Specific attention needs to be given to risk assessment, problem identification (whether physical, social, emotional or interpersonal) and support for the woman to maintain responsibility for her own safety, as well as that of her child

Maintenance and promotion of the physical health of the woman and infant. Specific attention may need to be given to individual activities of daily living, such as sleep, nutrition and personal hygiene

Facilitation of the development of emotional bonding between the mother and infant

Facilitation of the development of the parents' and family's communication and coping skills. The parents may need input to address practical childcare tasks, parenting and identification of additional sources of support

Provision of support for the mother and family. To address the stress associated with role change, personal and social expectations, and new family dynamics

---

The specific treatment approaches to perinatal mental health problems are similar to the medical and nursing management of the identified condition. The objectives of care during this period (Box 9.6) will be underpinned by the overall aim of ensuring the safety of the mother and child, with the principles of treatment focusing on the effective use of interpersonal skills, and attention to the woman's specific biological, psychological and social needs. Inherent are the skills of attending, listening and responding with empathy and a non-judgemental approach. Because of the huge emotional and physical adjustments that the woman and her family have to make during pregnancy and following childbirth, it is easy to unintentionally dismiss severe psychological distress. The importance of seeing each woman and her situation as unique is vital, as this way signs and symptoms of mental distress and ill health are less likely to be missed.

Many of the assessment and intervention skills required to deliver effective perinatal mental health care are already part of the midwife's and health visitor's skills set. The importance of the unique relationship that has been built up between the professional and the woman is the ideal platform for the delivery of specific interventions for mothers with mental health needs. While it can be tempting to see 'mental health' as the responsibility of others, the reality is that much mental health promotion and intervention can be effectively delivered by non-psychiatric staff. The role of specialist mental health workers may be more appropriately directed at activities such as staff education, liaison and clinical supervision. In this way the skills of these practitioners can be made available to a larger group of individuals than by utilising the traditional specialist referral, assessment and treatment model.

Conclusions

The perinatal period is an important stage in a woman's life and while it usually brings great joy and happiness, for some women and families it can bring the opposite. Women are more vulnerable during this period to developing a mental health problem or to experiencing a recurrence of an existing mental illness. However, service provision is inconsistent and communication between services has been consistently criticised for being poor. The woman may experience problems such as role conflict, difficulty in reconciling expectations to reality, and periods of fluctuating mood, all of which may precipitate more significant mental health difficulties. The experience of mental health problems can have an overwhelming effect on relationships and mothering, and tragically for a small minority, may even lead to death.

Midwives and health visitors have a pivotal role in mental health care during this period, being the lead maternity care providers and often having the closest contact with mothers and families. They should feel confident in their ability to detect vulnerability factors, screen for specific problems and make use of their close relationship and unique position to ensure that the communication and delivery of services for women at risk is given a high priority.

References

Beck, C. (2003) Postpartum depression screening scale. *Nursing Research*, 52 (5): 296–306.

Bewley, C. (2000) Postnatal depression. *Mental Health Practice*, 3 (7): 30–34.

Boath, E., Bradley, E. & Henshaw, C. (2004) Women's views of antidepressants in the treatment of postnatal depression. *Journal of Psychosomatic Obstetrics and Gynecology*, 25: 221–233.

Brockington, I.F. (1996) *Motherhood and Mental Health*. Oxford: Oxford University Press.

Brockington, I.F. (2004) Postpartum psychiatric disorders. *The Lancet*, 363: 303–310.

Buist, A.E., Barnett, B.E.W. & Milgrom, J. (2002) To screen or not to screen – that is the question in perinatal depression. *Medical Journal of Australia*, (Supplement) 177: S101–S105.

Burt, V.K., Suri, R. & Altshuler, L. (2001) The use of psychotropic medications during breast-feeding. *American Journal of Psychiatry*, 158: 1001–1009.

Clark, G. (2000) Discussing emotional health in pregnancy: the Edinburgh postnatal depression scale. *British Journal of Community Nursing*, 5: 91–98.

Cohen, L.S., Sichel, D.A. & Robertson, L.M. (1995) Postpartum prophylaxsis for women with bipolar disorder. *American Journal of Psychiatry*, 152: 1641–1645.

Confidential Enquiry into Maternal Deaths in the UK (2001) *Why Mothers Die – 1997–1999*. London: Royal College of General Practitioners Press.

Confidential Enquires into Maternal and Child Health (2004) *Why Mothers Die – 2000–2002*. London: Royal College of General Practitioners Press.

Cooper, P.J. & Murray, L. (1998) Postnatal depression: fortnightly review. *British Medical Journal*, 3161: 1259–1271.

Cox, J.L., Holden, J.M. & Sagovsky, R. (1987) Detection of postnatal depression. Development of the 10-item Edinburgh Postnatal Depression Scale. *British Journal of Psychiatry*, 150: 782–786.

Cox, J.L., Murray, D. & Chapman, G. (1993) A controlled study of the onset, duration and prevalence of postnatal depression. *British Journal of Psychiatry*, 163: 27–31.

Currid, T.J. (2004) Improving perinatal mental health care. *Nursing Standard*, 19 (3): 40–43.

Davies, B.R., Howells, S. & Jenkins, M. (2003) Early detection and treatment of postnatal depression in primary care. *Journal of Advanced Nursing*, 44 (3): 248–255.

Department of Health (1999) *National Service Framework for Mental Health*. London: DoH.

Department of Health (2003) *Mainstreaming Gender and Women's Mental Health: implementation guidance*. London: DoH.

Department of Health (2004) *National Service Framework for Children, Young People and Maternity Services*. London: DoH.

Evans, J., Heron, J. & Francomb, H. (2001) Cohort study of depressed mood during pregnancy and after childbirth. *British Medical Journal*, 323: 257–260.

Gaskell, C. (1999) A review of puerperal psychosis. *British Journal of Midwifery*, 7 (3): 172–174.

Green, J.M. (1998) Postnatal depression or perinatal dysphoria? Findings from a longitudinal community based study using the Edinburgh Postnatal Depression Scale. *Journal of Reproductive and Infant Psychology*, 16: 143–155.

Harvey, I. & McGrath, G. (1988) Psychiatric morbidity in spouses of women admitted to a mother and baby unit. *British Journal of Psychiatry*, 152: 506–510.

Hendrick, V. (2003) Treatment of postnatal depression. *British Medical Journal*, 327: 1003–1004.

Howard, L. (2000) Psychotic disorders and parenting – the relevance of patient's children for general adult psychiatric services. *Psychiatric Bulletin*, 24: 324–326.

Howard, L.M., Thornicroft, G. & Salmon, M. (2004) Predictors of parenting outcome in women with psychotic disorders discharged from mother and baby units. *Acta Psychiatrica Scandinavica*, 110 (5): 347–355.

Kacew, S. (1993) Adverse effects of drugs and chemicals in breast milk on the nursing infant. *Journal of Clinical Pharmacology*, 33: 213–221.

Kendell, R.E., Chalmer, J.C. & Platz, C. (1987) Epidemiology of puerperal psychosis. *British Journal of Psychiatry*, 150: 662–673.

Lee, D.T., Yip, A.S. & Chiu, H.F. (2000) Screening for postnatal depression using the double-test strategy. *Psychosomatic Medicine*, 62: 258–263.

Murray, L., Sinclair, D. & Cooper, P. (1999) The socioemotional development of 5 year old children of postnatally depressed mothers. *Journal of Child Psychology and Psychiatry*, 40: 1259–1271.

National Collaborating Centre for Women's and Children's Health (2003) *Antenatal Care: routine care for the healthy pregnant woman*. London: RCOG Press.

Nicholl, A. & Williams, A. (2002) Breast feeding. *Archives of Diseases in Childhood*, 87: 91–92.

Oates, M. (1996) Psychiatric services for women following childbirth. *International Review of Psychiatry*, 8: 87–98.

Price, S. (2004) Midwifery care and mental health. *Practising Midwife*, 7 (7): 12–14.

Royal College of Psychiatrists (2000) *Perinatal Mental Health Services*, (CR88), London: RCPsych.

Spigset, O. & Hågg, S. (1998) Excretion of psychotropic drugs into breast milk: pharmacokinetic overview and therapeutic implications. *CNS Drugs*, 9: 111–134.

Spigset, O. & Mårtensson, B. (1999) Drug treatment of depression. *British Medical Journal*, 318: 1188–1191.

Stein, G., Garth, D. & Butcher, J. (1991) The relationship between postnatal depression and mother–child interaction. *British Journal of Psychiatry*, 158: 46–52.

Chapter 10
Caring for the Person with a Serious Mental Illness

Chapter aims

> ### This chapter will:
>
> - describe the term 'serious mental illness' and identify those mental illnesses most commonly seen in the general hospital
> - describe the physical health problems associated with serious mental illness
> - discuss the factors influencing the identification, assessment and treatment of physical illness in this group of individuals
> - describe the principles of effective care planning for individuals with a serious mental illness who are being treated within the general hospital.

Introduction

While the number of patients with a serious mental illness (SMI) who are cared for within the general hospital at any one time is relatively small, they are nevertheless a group that deserve special attention. Co-existing medical illness and mental illness is common and those with an existing SMI receive less-than-adequate care when it comes to addressing their physical health care needs. This group of individuals is a heterogeneous group, and some people will cope relatively well with the experience of being unwell and of being admitted to hospital. However, others will require additional support and enhanced levels of nursing. This chapter will identify the core elements of effective care for this group of patients.

Definitions and terminology

There can be difficulty in achieving consistency in defining the term 'serious mental illness', although it is generally considered to be based on the following dimensions (Department of Health (DoH), 1996):

■ Safety/level of risk
■ Amount of informal and formal care required
■ Psychiatric diagnosis
■ Level of disability
■ Duration of illness.

It is generally accepted that the vast majority of individuals with an SMI will have a psychotic illness, characterised as a 'severe mental disorder in which the person's ability to recognise reality and his or her emotional responses, thinking processes, judgement and ability to communicate are so affected that his or her functioning is seriously impaired' (Warner, 1994). The illnesses most commonly allocated to this category are schizophrenia and bipolar affective disorder.

It is important to remember, however, that other psychiatric illnesses such as depression and anxiety can also be severely debilitating and have a major impact upon the person's lifestyle, relationships and social functioning. Whether or not such disorders are classified as 'serious' will be influenced by the nature and severity of symptoms, the duration of the disorder and the extent to which it has impacted on the person's life and ability to function independently.

An SMI will often follow a long-term course and the person's care is likely to be co-ordinated by the local community mental health team (CMHT). The *Care Programme Approach* (CPA) (DoH, 1990) was developed as a means of ensuring the effective delivery and co-ordination of care and treatment for people with an SMI. The CPA is aimed at ensuring that an assessment of need has been undertaken and an agreed care plan is in place, which is continually monitored (Armstrong, 1998). Importantly, this process requires that all individuals with an SMI are allocated a named mental health professional to act as their care co-ordinator.

Schizophrenia

Schizophrenia is a disorder that typically develops in late adolescence or early adulthood. It affects the sexes equally, but tends to be more severe and manifest at an earlier age in males. While the course of the illness varies, 25% of those experiencing a psychotic breakdown will recover without relapse, 50% will have another episode, and 25% will develop a severe and enduring mental illness (DoH, 1996). A useful framework for understanding schizophrenia involves separating the symptoms into 'positive' and 'negative'.

Positive symptoms are the most common and may include delusions and hallucinations, both of which can be the 'cause' of the apparently strange behaviour associated with the illness (Box 10.1).

Box 10.1 Understanding hallucinations and delusions.

Hallucinations

These are usually described as false sensory perceptions, or perceptual phenomena arising without any external stimulus, for example hearing (most common), seeing, smelling, feeling or tasting things that others do not. Some types of hallucination (e.g. visual) are common in the general population, but in those with an SMI, the voices will often be persecutory and critical in nature, or command the person to behave in a certain way. Hallucinations are described according to the sensory modality that they affect, and will be referred to as:

■ Auditory
■ Visual
■ Tactile
■ Gustatory
■ Olfactory

Delusions

A delusion is a false, firmly held belief that the person cannot be dissuaded from despite contradictory evidence. The belief is not based in the person's cultural, religious, educational or social experience and is maintained despite other members of the same culture not sharing it. For example, believing that there is the possibility of life elsewhere in the universe would be in keeping with the beliefs of many other people in society, but believing that the nurses on the ward are aliens would not be and would, thus, be a delusion.

A range of other 'psychotic phenomena' may also be present, including thought disorder or interference with thinking. This can result in conversation with the person being difficult, for example, it may appear to lack structure or purpose, or remain focused on the specific issue or idea that is causing distress for the person. At times the person may say that their thoughts have been inserted or removed from their mind, or believe that they are being broadcast to others.

Negative symptoms are less well known and as a result it can be assumed that they are a reflection of the person's personality, rather than as symptoms of the illness. Negative symptoms are more difficult to treat and tend to be present for a long time after the acute phase of the illness. They are often extremely distressing for the patient, family and significant others. Negative symptoms include:

■ *Blunted emotions.* Mood or affect appear 'flat', person shows little interest in everyday life, may seem socially withdrawn and uncommunicative.
■ *Cognitive deficits.* These impact on the person's ability to communicate, for

example, they will have difficulty in concentrating and will be slow to react to sensory input. These are often termed 'information-processing difficulties'.

■ *Apathy*. Difficulty undertaking straightforward tasks, with the person appearing slow and unmotivated.

Antipsychotic medication will be prescribed and usually has to be taken on a long-term basis. Medication is generally effective in treating the positive symptoms, but less so the negative ones. A combination of medication and social and psychological interventions, plus help and support to undertake specific activities of daily living, is the usual approach to treatment and clinical management.

Bipolar affective disorder

This is also referred to as 'manic depression', and is a cyclical disorder characterised by mood disturbances that consist of episodes of mania, depression or both. A diagnosis is fulfilled when the person has experienced two or more episodes of mania and two or more episodes of depression that last for at least one week and are severe enough to disrupt social and occupational functioning. These episodes must not be as a result of an organic cause, or linked to the use of substances, such as alcohol or illicit drugs (World Health Organization, 1992). Bipolar affective disorder affects between 1% and 2% of the population at some time in their lives and onset is usually before the age of 30 years, but can occur at any time. The most common pattern involves repeated episodes of mania or depression, usually followed by a period of remission. In severe mania, psychotic symptoms may also be present (Box 10.2).

During an episode of mania, the person is at risk of behaving in an antisocial way, possibly leading to serious financial, legal and relationship problems. The individual may well neglect their personal hygiene and physical health, and other psychiatric symptoms may be present (Table 10.1).

Box 10.2 Major symptoms of mania.

■ Elevated mood – characterised by grandiose ideas and inflated self-esteem
■ Increased energy and activity
■ Increased creativity
■ Increased sociability
■ Increased libido
■ Decreased need to sleep
■ Impaired concentration and attention
■ Flight of ideas – when thoughts race through the mind more quickly than they can be expressed

Table 10.1 Psychiatric symptoms seen in serious mental illness.

	Delusions	Hallucinations	Thought disorder
Schizophrenia	♦♦♦	♦♦♦	♦♦♦
Bipolar affective disorder	♦♦	♦♦	♦♦
Depression	♦♦	♦	♦

Often ♦♦♦ Sometimes ♦♦ Rarely ♦

Mortality and morbidity associated with serious mental illness

Those suffering from an SMI experience increased rates of morbidity and mortality (Brown, 1997). This association has been known for a long time, yet relatively little has been written on the physical care of people with SMI in the general hospital. People with schizophrenia are between two and four times more likely to die prematurely than a person in the general population, with an average lifespan at least ten years shorter than their age-related counterparts (Goldman, 2000). People with SMI are at risk of developing a number of physical health problems and illnesses, the reasons for which are complex and multi-factorial (Table 10.2).

Factors that contribute to poor physical health

A number of factors are associated with poor physical health in people with an SMI, including:

- *Social factors*, e.g. poverty, unemployment, social isolation and exclusion, poor access to and uptake of mainstream health care services, such as primary care, dental services, ophthalmology, personal health and lifestyle facilities (gyms, leisure centres, etc.).
- *Psychological factors*, e.g. low self-esteem, lack of personal assertiveness.
- *Illness-related factors*, e.g. side effects and iatrogenic complications of medication used to treat SMI.
- *Personal factors*, e.g. higher rates of smoking, lack of physical exercise.
- *Professional factors*, e.g. health staff less likely to offer preventive health care, lack of 'ownership' for the physical health of people with SMI from both primary care and mental health staff (Jones, 2004).

The issue of smoking is discussed below to illustrate the overlap of the various factors described above. Eighty per cent of people with schizophrenia smoke and research has shown that death from respiratory disease is one of the most common causes of mortality (Brown *et al.*, 2000). Smoking also impairs the effectiveness of antipsychotic medication. As a group, these

Table 10.2 Physical health problems and illnesses associated with serious mental illness.

Problem/illness	Comments
Cardiovascular disorders	Increased incidence of cardiovascular disorders associated with schizophrenia (Herman *et al.*, 1983); adverse effects of medication and lifestyle issues are thought to play a part
Gastrointestinal disorders	Increased rate of peptic ulceration, gastrointestinal and pancreatic cancers, and irritable bowel syndrome (Newman & Bland, 1991; Jeste *et al.*, 1996). The higher use of alcohol in people with SMI is thought to be a contributory factor
Neurological disorders	Co-morbid neurological symptoms are common – contributory factors include, higher rate of head injuries, pre-natal trauma and excessive alcohol use. Antipsychotics reduce seizure thresholds and excessive alcohol increases vulnerability to seizures. Long-term use of antipsychotics can cause neurological complications, including dystonia and tardive dyskinesia (Mirza & Phelan, 2002) (see Table 10.3)
Endocrine disorders	People with schizophrenia are more likely to develop type 2 diabetes than the general population, although the reasons are not clear. Insulin resistance may be a factor, as well as the effects of antipsychotic medication, which tends to induce glucose intolerance (Pomeroy *et al.*, 2002)
Infections	Increased risk of developing tuberculosis (TB), human immunodeficiency virus (HIV) and hepatitis C. Those with an SMI may be at risk of engaging in behaviours, such as intravenous drug use and higher risk sexual activity, that increase the risk of acquiring such infections (Brunette *et al.*, 1999)
Musculoskeletal disorders	Antipsychotic medication, particularly when prescribed for older people, can cause postural hypotension, leading to falls and fractures. Higher incidence of osteoporosis in people with schizophrenia (Goldman, 2000)
Respiratory disorders	High rates of emphysema and recurrent chest infections probably associated with higher rates of cigarette smoking. Increased risk of mortality in people with asthma who are prescribed antipsychotics (Joseph *et al.*, 1996)

individuals are less likely to receive advice on the harmful effects of smoking and the benefits of smoking cessation. Mental health staff are more likely to smoke than other health professionals (Dore & Hoey, 1988) and smoking is often seen as more acceptable as 'It's their only pleasure'. Despite more positive public health policy approaches to smoking cessation in the general population, there is a view that smoking cessation for someone with an SMI will exacerbate their mental illness. For many, it is seen as a coping mechanism for dealing with psychological and emotional distress. Furthermore, the stigma associated with mental ill health may lead others to believe that these individuals will not be able to persevere and manage to stop smoking completely, yet there is growing evidence as to the effectiveness of smoking cessation programmes for people with SMI (George *et al.*, 2002).

Assessment

Individuals who suffer from an SMI require a comprehensive assessment of their biological, psychological and social needs, as all of these areas will have an influence on assessment and care planning. Some important factors that may act as a barrier to effective assessment include:

- Communication difficulties, possibly due to fear, anxiety, depression or cognitive impairment.
- Presence of co-morbid conditions, such as excessive alcohol use.
- Co-morbid medical conditions – these may become 'masked' or overlooked, assuming that symptoms are a result of the person's mental illness, rather than their physical condition.
- Generally poor physical health, such as poor nutrition, poor oral hygiene, or obesity.

Nurses engaged in the assessment process will need to make every effort to develop an effective rapport with the person – a process that is enhanced if attention is given to specific aspects of communication and collaboration (Box 10.3).

Achieving co-operation and concordance between the patient and the care team is vital, although it has long been known that a large percentage of medical illnesses are either undiagnosed or poorly treated in people with an existing mental illness (Pomeroy *et al.*, 2002). Specifically in patients with an SMI it has been found that fewer medical diagnoses are made, they are

---

Box 10.3 Factors that enhance the communication and engagement processes.

- Knowing something of the person's background and history
- Conferring and liaising with the local CMHT involved in the person's care
- Using contact as a means of getting to know the person
- Explaining factual information in clear, straightforward language and checking for understanding. Information may have to be repeated several times
- Consulting with relatives and carers – utilising their input in the care planning and delivery processes

admitted more frequently and are treated later in the acute phase of their illness (Lamden *et al.*, 1997). Specific factors that will impact on the ability of the nurse to develop a rapport with the person and thereby form an accurate picture of their nursing needs are:

- *Patient factors.* The symptoms of an SMI are not viewed as part of the illness process, consequently, the patient may be thought of as being 'difficult' and unmotivated to help him or herself. If positive symptoms such as hallucinations and delusions are exhibited, these can appear bizarre and frightening for staff. Suspicion and paranoid thinking may also make it difficult to engage with the person, resulting in only cursory assessment or examination and a premature or inaccurate diagnosis (Vieweg *et al.*, 1995). Finally, the patient may have difficulty in reporting and describing symptoms, so their account lacks detail and can appear 'unreliable'.
- *Staff factors.* People with mental health problems report feeling discriminated against by health care staff, including staff in the general hospital, with a common complaint being that their physical illnesses are not taken seriously (Mental Health Foundation, 2000). A diagnosis of SMI can evoke high levels of anxiety in staff, influenced by their previous experience, lack of knowledge and training, as well as a perceived lack of professional skills. Added to this is the fact that caring for a person with an SMI requires them to use their patient-contact time in a different way. This is something that many find challenging and difficult, and is reinforced by the negative and stereotypical belief that this group of patients are unrewarding to care for.
- *Diagnostic difficulties.* It may be difficult at times to distinguish between the symptoms of mental illness and the psychological presentation of complications of medical illness. This is compounded by the fact that a number of medical illnesses can present with primary psychiatric symptoms, and the side effects of various medications can mimic psychiatric symptoms. (See also Chapters 2 and 7.)

Pharmacological treatment of serious mental illness

Antipsychotic medication

Antipsychotic medication is used as treatment in the acute phase and long-term management of psychotic illnesses such as schizophrenia. These drugs have been shown to reduce the relapse rate and are effective in treating positive symptoms. They are divided into various groups according to the individual drug's chemical structure or potency. Their antipsychotic action is attributed to their anti-dopaminergic activity. Second generation antipsychotics have been developed and are termed 'atypical', as opposed to the original, first generation drugs. An understanding of this is important as the side effect profile of the two groups differs (Box 10.4).

Box 10.4 Side effects of antipsychotic medication.

First generation antipsychotics

■ Anticholinergic effects – blurred vision, dry mouth, constipation, urinary retention, memory and cognitive impairments, hallucinations
■ Extrapyramidal side effects

Second generation (atypical) antipsychotics

■ Haematological side effects – including agranulocytosis (clozapine)
■ Increased risk of type 2 diabetes, ketoacidosis and pancreatitis
■ Affect lipid metabolism – increase in serum triglycerides

All antipsychotics

■ Cardiovascular effects – some can cause postural hypotension and ECG changes, in particular increased Q-T interval
■ Metabolic and endocrine problems – hyperprolactinaemia, type 2 diabetes
■ Sedation
■ Weight gain
■ Sexual dysfunction, linked to hyperprolactinaemia, e.g. galactorrhoea, erectile difficulties and/or ejaculation problems, menstrual irregularities, gynaecomastia in men
■ Hepatic side effects
■ Lower seizure threshold

Extrapyramidal side effects (EPSEs) are often overlooked or mistaken as symptoms of agitation and, to the unaware, can be mistaken as part of the underlying illness (Table 10.3). It is important to remember that EPSEs also occur with medically prescribed drugs that have anti-dopaminergic properties, such as metaclopramide.

Use of atypical antipsychotics has been shown to lead to positive outcomes for a number of patients and they are generally associated with fewer overall side effects than the first generation antipsychotics. Examples of 'atypicals' include:

■ Amisulpride
■ Clozapine
■ Olanzapine
■ Quetiapine
■ Risperidone
■ Zotepine.

These drugs are recommended as first line treatment in people with newly diagnosed schizophrenia (National Institute for Clinical Excellence, 2002). Clozapine has side effects that could precipitate a medical admission and it cannot simply be discontinued or restarted at previous doses. Its use is also contraindicated in a variety of medical conditions.

Table 10.3 Extrapyramidal side effects of antipsychotic medication.

Side effect	Characterised by	Treatment
Parkinsonism	Shuffling gait Tremor Muscle stiffness Limb 'cog wheeling'	Responds to dose reduction or treatment with an anticholinergic drug such as procyclidine
Dystonia	Involuntary muscular contraction	Responds to dose reduction or treatment with an anticholinergic drug such as procyclidine
Akathesia	Subjective or inner feeling of restlessness	Responds to dose reduction and treatment with propanolol or clonazepam Anticholinergics are only effective if parkinsonism is also present
Tardive dyskinesia (TD)	Involuntary movements of the mouth, lips and tongue, which may progress to the head, neck and trunk. This is most likely to be seen as a result of long-term treatment	Dose reduction or treatment with anticholinergics may worsen TD. As treatment is complex, contact specialist mental health staff, ward pharmacist and local drug information service. TD has been known to affect muscles of the respiratory and gastrointestinal systems

Mood stabilisers

Mood stabilisers are used in the treatment of bipolar affective disorder and include:

- Lithium carbonate
- Carbamazepine
- Sodium valproate.

Lithium is a first line treatment and is often given in conjunction with antipsychotic medication if the person has psychotic features to their illness. It has a narrow therapeutic index and optimal serum lithium concentration needs to be within the range of 0.40–1.00 mmol/l. Outside this, a lower level will be ineffective and indicative of a high risk of relapse, while if the level rises above the therapeutic range, toxicity can occur. Concentrations in excess of 2.00 mmol/l can be potentially fatal. Risk factors for developing lithium toxicity are conditions leading to sodium depletion, for example, diarrhoea, vomiting and excessive sweating. Medication that reduces renal excretion of lithium, such as thiazide diuretics and certain non-steroidal anti-inflammatory drugs can also lead to toxicity.

If a person is admitted to hospital with an acute medical illness, a baseline serum lithium level should be taken. The signs and symptoms of acute lithium toxicity are:

- Nausea, diarrhoea, vomiting
- Severe tremor, ataxia, slurred speech, choreiform and parkinsonian movements, muscular twitching, seizures
- Impaired concentration, drowsiness, disorientation.

Treatment should be discontinued and serum lithium and urea and electrolytes monitored. The provision of adequate salt and fluids, including saline infusions, will reduce toxicity. Caution is needed when prescribing lithium to individuals with renal failure, heart failure, recent myocardial infarction, electrolyte imbalance, and to pregnant women and older people.

As a general rule, if a person is admitted to hospital and is currently receiving psychotropic medication, this should be continued during medical and surgical treatment (Kruk *et al.*, 1995). There will obviously be exceptions to this in certain situations, for example, if the medication is specifically contra-indicated in patients with specific medical conditions, or when potentially serious drug interactions may occur as a result of newly instigated treatment. If they are currently receiving antipsychotic medication by intra-muscular injection (depot injection), the ward team should ascertain the frequency and details of when it is next due, as well as any other individual patient needs associated with its administration. In order to clarify these points it will be necessary to make contact with the named nurse who usually administers the medication – this may be the patient's community psychiatric nurse (CPN) or the practice nurse if the patient normally attends a primary care facility.

Principles of caring for a person with a serious mental illness

Admission to hospital is likely to be a stressful event for all patients (see Chapter 2), in particular because the environment is novel and is often perceived as unpredictable and uncontrollable. People with an SMI may find it harder than others to tolerate and cope with sudden and unfamiliar events, possibly producing a maladaptive response which can result in a worsening of their psychiatric symptoms. Developing an effective rapport and relationship with the person can help minimise the stressful impact of the hospital experience and is a key nursing priority (Box 10.5).

On admission efforts must be made to reduce the stress associated with a new environment. Welcoming the patient, offering regular short discussions to orientate them to the ward, explaining the 'routine' and what is likely to happen to them, will all help to reduce levels of stress and anxiety.

Box 10.5 Benefits of developing effective rapport and relationship.

■ Ensures that you are more likely to gain an accurate picture of what the real health or illness problems are for the person, e.g. medical diagnosis is more likely to be accurate
■ Individual is more likely to accept the treatment and care offered and to continue it long term
■ Person is more likely to be satisfied with their care and less likely to feel distressed and ignored
■ Reduces the risk of the person exhibiting behavioural distress that can be associated with increased stress, fear and uncertainty

---

Specific symptoms require targeted interpersonal responses, for example, problems with memory can be addressed by offering reminders, providing written information and checking the person's understanding. The nurse needs to demonstrate empathy and use active listening skills, as well as showing a degree of patience and perseverance when communicating. There also needs to be a willingness to understand the person, valuing their views and opinions, and a significant element of nursing care will hinge on the ability to deliver patient-focused interventions in a sensitive way (Table 10.4). A major requirement is to ensure that the patient is given adequate time to express his needs, while recognising that this can be challenging in a busy clinical environment. If adequate attention is not given to this, it is likely that the person will not fully understand the care and treatment being offered. Complications and further difficulties can then ensue, which will prove even more costly in terms of time.

Liaison and joint working with the person's care co-ordinator (e.g. CPN or social worker) from the local CMHT is essential to aid assessment, treatment and nursing care. They will be able to supply information and advice on the best approaches to use when communicating with the person, as well as contribute to the development of a comprehensive care plan. If there are specific difficulties or problems identified, then the CMHT care co-ordinator should be asked to take the lead in working with the patient and the hospital team in order to overcome these. On discharge the CMHT should be fully involved in all aftercare and follow-up arrangements. They may have to take a central role in ensuring a co-ordinated approach from primary and secondary care in meeting the person's needs once discharged. The role of the patient's partner, relatives and carers needs to be incorporated into the discharge planning process at an early stage.

Finally, at an organisational level, training is required to increase hospital nurses' confidence and competence in working with people who have an SMI, supported by ongoing clinical supervision. These are vitally important elements in fostering a positive attitude towards this group of patients, which in turn, assists nurses to provide holistic and effective care.

Table 10.4 Core nursing interventions for the person experiencing acute symptoms of a serious mental illness.

Intervention	Rationale
Ensure evaluation of mental state as part of nursing assessment	Provides a baseline against which to assess improvement or deterioration
Use non-judgemental and non-critical responses; offer reassurance and demonstrate acceptance	Reduces the stress associated with alterations in thinking and perception
Maintain regular social contact – do not avoid the person or isolate them within the ward	Isolating and avoiding the person is likely to increase feelings of anxiety and suspicion
Use clear straightforward language, e.g. avoid jargon, approach unhurriedly, maintain eye contact and open posture. Avoid overt criticism and negative comments, accept apparently 'one-sided' or bizarre conversations	Ensures that communication is clear and unambiguous. Reduces the likelihood of the person displaying apparently unco-operative or 'difficult' behaviours
Reassure the person that they are safe within the ward, and of your non-harmful intent	Can act to reduce suspicious thoughts and anxious feelings
Maintain accurate record of the person's verbal and non-verbal behaviour, e.g. angry, hallucinating, impulsive, irritable, withdrawn, dietary and fluid intake	Enables any improvements or deterioration in symptomatology to be monitored and evaluated. Ensures that physical health needs are met
If the person is disturbed or agitated, refrain from unnecessary actions or procedures	These may increase feelings of anxiety and suspicious thoughts
If possible and practicable, involve the person's partner/carer/significant other in the assessment and delivery of care	Can provide reassurance and consistency in care delivery and helps maintain a vital link to the person's usual routine

Conclusions

People with an SMI experience relatively high rates of physical ill health, some of which are as a direct consequence of their illness and its treatment, and some of which are associated with societal factors such as the stigma, ignorance, fear and stereotypical attitudes towards those with mental illness. All professionals need to adopt a more proactive role in addressing the health and treatment needs of this group. This chapter has highlighted some of the health and illness problems associated with SMI and has identified the role that general hospital nurses can play in improving both the individual's health and their experience of hospital when they are physically unwell.

Ensuring effective assessment and treatment for people with an SMI and co-morbid medical illness within the general hospital is a challenging task, and nurses need to be aware of the needs of this group of patients and how to plan and deliver care that meets physical, emotional and social needs. Effective care primarily depends upon forming an effective relationship and close collaboration with the patient, their relatives and carers, as well as good liaison and collaborative working between the hospital-based team and the CMHT.

References

Armstrong, E. (1998) The primary/secondary care interface. In: C. Brooker & J. Repper (eds), *Serious Mental Health Problems in the Community: policy and research*, pp. 87–108. London: Baillière Tindall.

Brown, S. (1997) Excessive mortality of schizophrenia. *British Journal of Psychiatry*, 171: 502–508.

Brown, S., Inksip, H. & Barrowclough, B. (2000) Causes of excess mortality in schizophrenia. *British Journal of Psychiatry*, 177: 212–217.

Brunette, M.F., Rosenberg, S.D. & Goodman, L.A. (1999) HIV risk factors among people with severe mental illness in urban and rural areas. *Psychiatric Services*, 50: 556–558.

Department of Health (1990) *Care Programme Approach*. London: HMSO.

Department of Health (1996) *The Health of the Nation: building bridges*. London: HMSO.

Dore, K. & Hoey, J. (1988) Smoking practices: knowledge and attitudes regarding smoking of university hospital nurses. *Canadian Journal of Public Health*, 79: 170–174.

George, T.P., Vessiochio, J.C. & Termine, A. (2002) A placebo controlled trial of bupropion for smoking cessation in schizophrenia. *Biological Psychiatry*, 52 (1): 53–61.

Goldman, L.S. (2000) Co-morbid medical illness in psychiatric patients. *Current Psychiatry Reports*, 2: 236–263.

Herman, H.E., Baldwin, J.A. & Christie, D. (1983) A record-linkage study of mortality and general hospital discharge in patients diagnosed as schizophrenic. *Psychological Medicine*, 13: 581–598.

Jeste, D.V., Gladsjo, J.A. & Lindamer, L.A. (1996) Medical co-morbidity in schizophrenia. *Schizophrenia Bulletin*, 22: 412–430.

Jones, A. (2004) Mind over matter: physical wellbeing for people with severe mental illness. *Mental Health Practice*, 7 (10): 36–38.

Joseph, K.S., Blais, L. & Singh, S. (1996) Increased morbidity and mortality related to asthma among asthmatic patients that use major tranquilisers. *British Medical Journal*, 3112: 79–82.

Kruk, J., Sachdev, P. & Singh, S. (1995) Neuroleptic induced respiratory dyskinesia. *Journal of Neuropsychiatry and Clinical Neuroscience*, 7: 223–229.

Lamden, R.M., Ramchondani, D. & Schindler, B.A. (1997) The chronically mentally ill in a general hospital: consultation liaison service. *Psychosomatics*, 38: 472–477.

Mental Health Foundation (2000) *Pull Yourself Together: a survey of the stigma and discrimination faced by people who experience mental distress*. London: MHF.

Mirza, L. & Phelan, M. (2002) Managing physical illness in people with severe mental illness. *Hospital Medicine*, 63 (9): 535–539.

National Institute for Clinical Excellence (2002) *Guidance On the Use of Newer (Atypical) Antipsychotic Drugs for the Treatment of Schizophrenia*. London: NICE.

Newman, S.C. & Bland, R.C. (1991) Mortality in a cohort of patients with schizophrenia: a record-linkage study. *Canadian Journal of Psychiatry*, 36: 229–245.

Pomeroy, C., Mitchell, J.E. & Roeng, J. (2002) *Medical Complications of Psychiatric Illness*. Arlington: American Psychiatric Publishing.

Vieweg, V., Levenson, J. & Pendurang, A. (1995) Medical disorders in the schizophrenic patient. *International Journal of Psychiatry in Medicine*, 25 (2): 137–172.

Warner, R. (1994) *Recovery from Schizophrenia: psychiatry and political economy*. London: Routledge.

World Health Organization (1992) *International Classification of Impairments, Disabilities and Handicaps*. Geneva: WHO.

Chapter 11
Alcohol and Illicit Drug Use

Chapter aims

> ### This chapter will:
>
> - describe the prevalence of alcohol and drug-related health problems within the general hospital
> - describe the screening and assessment of individuals with suspected alcohol and drug use problems
> - discuss the presentation and treatment of alcohol and opiate withdrawal
> - identify the treatment and clinical management strategies that can be used when caring for the person with an alcohol or drug-related problem
> - discuss the nurse's role in relation to health promotion and encouraging personal change.

Introduction

The presentation of patients who use excessive amounts of alcohol and/or illicit drugs (in this chapter drug misuse refers to the use of illicit/illegal/ street drugs) is of growing concern to staff working in a general hospital setting.

The rates of excessive alcohol and drug use are markedly higher in hospitalised medical and surgical patients (and in patients with psychiatric disorders and mental illness) than in the general population (Allen *et al.*, 1998). Use of these substances is a major cause of attendance both to emergency departments (EDs) and non-emergency clinical settings. They can be the primary reason for admission or attendance, for example, acute alcohol intoxication, or may be a causative factor underlying other medical or surgical presentations, for example, an infected injection site in a person who uses intravenous drugs. Alcohol use may be responsible for at least 10% of hospital attendances and a large proportion of head and facial injuries and trauma (Royal College of Physicians, 2001), and it is reported that one in six people attending the ED for treatment have alcohol-related injuries or problems, which rises to a staggering eight in ten at peak times (Waller *et al.*, 1998).

Definitions and terminology

Like other psychiatric conditions, the diagnosis of alcohol and drug misuse is outlined by the World Health Organization (WHO) (2003) in the *International Classification of Mental and Behavioural Disorders* (ICD-10). A diagnosis is made when there is a mental and behavioural problem due to the use of alcohol or drugs, for example, excessive alcohol consumption or use of illicit opioids (the range of drugs misused is discussed later in this chapter).

Alcohol and drug misuse is defined as the excessive use of that substance, although in clinical practice it must be remembered that polysubstance (multiple substances) use is often the norm. Use of the substances described in this chapter can all lead to dependency, potentially resulting in physical or emotional harm, and may be the underlying cause of a range of social and interpersonal problems, such as employment and relationship difficulties. With repeated use of substances tolerance can develop, so that the person has to take more of the substance to achieve the desired effect. Stopping using the substance may lead to a state of withdrawal, manifesting both physical and psychological symptoms. For clinical management reasons alone it is important that the nurse has a good understanding of the terms outlined above, specifically:

- *Acute intoxication.* Caused by excessive use.
- *Harmful use.* A pattern of misuse that is causing damage to health, for example, hepatitis from the re-use of contaminated injecting equipment.
- *Dependency syndrome.* Develops after repeated use that leads to increased physiological and psychological tolerance.
- *Withdrawal state.* Development of a group of symptoms (dependent upon the type and amount of substance used) due to the sudden cessation or marked reduction in the amount of substance used.

Acute intoxication

This follows the use of psychoactive substances such as alcohol or heroin, and results in altered consciousness, impaired cognition, altered perception and out-of-character behaviour (e.g. disinhibition), or changes to other psycho-physiological functions and responses. It occurs as a result of the acute pharmacological effect of the substance and resolves in time with complete recovery, except where specific complications have arisen, for example, trauma or inhalation of vomit (Box 11.1).

> **Box 11.1** Summary of the physiological and psychological effects of acute alcohol intoxication and acute opioid intoxication (WHO, 1992).
>
> - Disinhibition
> - Argumentativeness
> - Aggression
> - Lability of mood
> - Impaired attention
> - Impaired judgement
> - Interference with personal functioning
>
> Other signs that may be present include:
>
> - Unsteady gait
> - Difficulty in standing
> - Slurred speech
> - Nystagmus
> - Decreased level of consciousness, e.g. stupor, coma
> - Flushed face
> - Conjunctival infection

Harmful use

This is a pattern of psychoactive substance use that is causing damage to health. Although the focus here is on the physical and psychological impact of such use, it must be remembered that any excessive use of substances will have marked social and interpersonal consequences. Harm can be associated with acute intoxication and hazardous use, for instance, consuming excessive amounts of alcohol over the course of a week, or drinking excessive amounts in a single session (termed binge drinking).

Unlike illicit drug use (which is illegal), a degree of alcohol use is generally accepted as the norm in Western society, with the vast majority of the UK population consuming alcohol to some degree. This is not to say that concerns are not raised about its use, whether this is for health or social reasons. The UK Alcohol Forum (2001) states that a safe level of alcohol consumption is a misnomer, as no level of alcohol is totally devoid of risk. It also states that alcohol-free days are important for good health. Recently, however, research has begun to suggest that light to moderate drinking is associated with a reduced risk of coronary heart disease and ischaemic stroke, as well as improved overall mortality in middle-aged and elderly people (Agarwal, 2002). However, this apparent benefit in relation to heart disease mortality is offset by higher alcohol consumption increasing the risk of death from other types of heart disease, such as cardiomyopathy and arrhythmias.

The medical royal colleges, including the Royal College of Physicians, have all recommended that men should drink less than 21 units of alcohol per week and women less than 14 units per week (Box 11.2). Advice from the Department of Health (DoH) (1995) refers to increased morbidity and mortality associated with drinking more than three to four units a day for men and two

> **Box 11.2** Definition of a unit of alcohol (Royal College of Physicians, 2001).
>
> A 'unit' contains 8 g of alcohol. This is approximately the amount of alcohol contained in:
>
> ■ Half of a pint (approximately 300 ml) of ordinary strength beer or cider
> ■ Quarter of a pint (approximately 150 ml) of extra strong beer or cider
> ■ A small (100 ml) glass of wine, sherry or port
> ■ A single measure (25 ml) of spirits

to three units for women. This advice may lead to some confusion, as it implicitly implies an increased weekly limit above that recommended by the UK Alcohol Forum (2001). It is important to appreciate that harm can result not only when the person is alcohol dependent but also as a result of hazardous use. These guidelines are based on research into the relationship between alcohol and disease in adults and cannot be assumed to apply to children and adolescents, adults who have specific health problems or pregnant women.

The physiological and pharmacokinetic effects of alcohol are influenced by factors such as gender, body weight and the rate and amount of alcohol consumed. In order to reach the same blood level concentration, a greater amount of alcohol will generally be required by a heavier person than one of lower body weight.

Virtually every system in the human body can be damaged by alcohol (Royal College of Physicians, 2001). There are also health complications associated with illicit drug use and these can be attributed to the type of drug use, the technique used to administer the drug and the person's lifestyle (Table 11.1 and Box 11.3).

Individuals who use excessive amount of alcohol or use illicit drugs are at increased risk of psychological problems. Both can impair judgement, decision-making, as well as increase levels of impulsiveness. This can lead to antisocial and disinhibited behaviour, such as engaging in violent or criminal activity.

Dependency

This can develop after repeated and long-term alcohol use. With illicit drugs it can occur after even short-term use. The phenomenon of dependency includes the following characteristics:

■ a strong desire to consume the substance
■ difficulty in controlling and limiting its use
■ persisting in its use despite being aware of and experiencing harmful consequences
■ the individual gives a high priority to taking or obtaining the substance over other activities and personal obligations
■ development of tolerance – the need to take increasing amounts to produce the same desired effect, or a marked diminished effect with continued use of the same amount.

Table 11.1 The health and medical complications of excessive alcohol use.

Body system	Complication
Gastrointestinal	Cirrhosis of liver, hepatitis
	Gastritis
	Pancreatitis
	Gastrointestinal haemorrhage
	Malnutrition, weight loss, malabsorption
Cardiovascular	Cardiac arrhythmias
	Cardiomyopathy
	Hypertension – often difficult to treat
Neurological	Blackouts
	Convulsions
	Peripheral neuropathy
	Acute confusional states
	Head injuries
	Long-term brain damage
	Depression
Respiratory	Pneumonia – inhalation of vomit while intoxicated
Reproductive	Men
	Hypogonadism – loss of libido, impotence, loss of secondary sexual characteristics, gynaecomastia
	Infertility
	Women
	Hypogonadism – loss of libido, menstrual irregularities, loss of secondary sexual characteristics
Musculoskeletal	Gout
Other	Increased risk of certain cancers, in particular of the mouth, oesophagus, liver and colon
	Increased incidence of alcohol-related trauma
	Increased risk of self-harm and suicide

Withdrawal

This is a group of symptoms that occur following sudden total or reduced withdrawal of the substance after its persistent use. The onset, course and symptoms of the withdrawal are time limited and related to the type and dosage of the substance. Admission to hospital is an event that will precipitate the sudden cessation of previous alcohol or drug use, and may require measures to prevent the manifestations of acute withdrawal symptoms.

It is important to be aware of the symptoms of withdrawal across the range of substances commonly used. Specific attention should be given to the withdrawal symptoms of alcohol (Box 11.4) and opioids (Table 11.2). If the person is experiencing acute alcohol or opiate withdrawal, then supportive treatment will need to be given while the person is in hospital. The symptoms and complications of withdrawal may be relatively minor, but

Box 11.3 The health and medical complications of illicit drug use (Crowe *et al.*, 2000; Pomeroy, 2002).

Complications arising from needle sharing and contaminants used include:

- Serious soft tissue infections, e.g. cellulitis, abscesses
- Thrombophlebitis
- Deep venous thrombosis
- Infective endocarditis
- Septicaemia
- Hepatitis
- Arterial puncture
- Increased risk of human immune deficiency virus (HIV) transmission and acquired immune deficiency syndrome (AIDS)
- Gangrene

Respiratory complications include pneumonia and increased rate of tuberculosis (TB). There is a link between communicable disease transmission and those who use illicit substances

Higher rates of liver and renal disease

Dietary complications, e.g. weight loss, malnutrition, constipation

Increased risk of self-harm and suicide

Box 11.4 Symptoms of acute alcohol withdrawal.

Early symptoms – may be classed as 'minor':

- Coarse tremor of the hands, tongue, eyelids
- Stomach 'cramps', abdominal discomfort, loss of appetite
- Paroxysmal sweats
- Tachycardia
- Insomnia
- Irritability

If untreated, more severe symptoms can include:

- Disorientation
- Confusion
- Perceptual disturbance – most commonly visual hallucinations – 'seeing things', possibly insects or spiders
- Marked tachycardia
- Profuse sweating and flushed appearance

If untreated, withdrawal can progress to delirium tremens (DT), which can involve marked psychomotor agitation, seizures, coma and death. Seizures can occur as early as six hours after the last drink, with the peak risk period being within the first 48 hours. All individuals with a history of seizures should be managed in hospital during initial withdrawal from alcohol

Table 11.2 Symptoms of acute opiate withdrawal.

Withdrawal from opiates is not life threatening, although subjectively very unpleasant	
Subjective symptoms	Drug craving
	Restlessness
	Low mood
	Irritability
	Fatigue
	Hot and cold flushes
	Appetite loss
	Aching muscles and joints
	Nausea
	Abdominal discomfort and cramps
Objective signs	Dilated pupils
	Sweating
	Tremor
	Diarrhoea
	Rhinorrhoea
	Vomiting
	Tachycardia
	Sneezing
	Hypertension
	Frequent yawning
	Lacrimation
	Pyrexia

they can also become so severe that they warrant urgent medical treatment. Opiate withdrawal, although subjectively unpleasant, rarely leads to serious complications, whereas untreated acute alcohol withdrawal can be fatal.

Some substances, such as cocaine, amphetamines, cannabis and solvents can all be discontinued abruptly without significant physical withdrawal symptoms, and there is no recommended substitution treatment for these drugs (Ashworth & Gerada, 1997). Benzodiazepines, although usually prescribed drugs, can also be obtained and used illicitly, have an associated physical withdrawal state and therefore if a patient is admitted on benzodiazepines these should normally be continued during their hospital stay. If benzodiazepines or hypnotics are initiated during hospital admission, these should not be continued beyond the time limits set in the *British National Formulary*, usually between two to four weeks maximum.

Commonly misused illicit drugs

Common drugs of misuse tend to cause euphoria and an increased sense of pleasure (Ashworth & Gerada, 1997). Stimulants are typically amphetamines and cocaine, chronic use of which can lead to paranoia, anxiety and panic, as opposed to the euphoria of early use (Kushner, 1991). The physical signs of intoxication from stimulants include tachycardia, hypertension, increased respiratory rate and increased body temperature. If the level of ingestion is high, seizures and cardiovascular collapse can occur. Opiates, in particular heroin, produce an intense but transient feeling of pleasure and euphoria, followed by sedation.

Hallucinogenics are typically lysergic acid diethylamide (LSD), hallucinogenic mushrooms and cannabis. LSD is associated with perceptual disturbances rather than frank hallucinations. Intoxication is usually characterised by mild signs of autonomic arousal such as tachycardia and pupillary dilation. Protecting the person from harm and 'talking them down' is usually sufficient management of intoxication.

Ecstasy, also known as E, has hallucinogenic properties and produces euphoria and increased energy. Excessive use causes raised physical activity and can lead to death through hyperthermia and dehydration (Ashworth & Gerada, 1997).

Assessment

Patients can be admitted to hospital specifically for their alcohol or drug problem, for instance, if they are presenting in an intoxicated state, or they experience acute withdrawal symptoms. It is important for the practitioner to recognise the condition and ensure appropriate treatment and monitoring is undertaken.

The majority of patients with alcohol and drug-related problems will be in hospital for a specific medical or surgical reason that may not appear to be directly connected to their underlying alcohol or drug problem, for example, heart disease or trauma. Due to the high prevalence of alcohol and drug-related presentations within general hospitals, it is advocated that all patients are screened for usage and a more in-depth assessment conducted as required. The rationale for this approach is that it will increase the likelihood of the identification of underlying substance use problems and will benefit the patient by ensuring that:

- any treatment required for withdrawal or maintenance treatment can be instigated, e.g. prompt management of withdrawal
- appropriate clinical management will increase the likelihood of the patient accepting treatment for their medical condition
- opportunities for health promotion and harm reduction interventions are provided
- the person is helped to gain insight into their harmful behaviour and make informed choices regarding seeking further help to change their lifestyle.

All patients should be asked about alcohol and drug use as part of a routine nursing assessment. It is important to demonstrate empathy and to adopt a non-judgemental or non-confrontational attitude, thereby ensuring that their alcohol or drug use is not viewed negatively and that their right to appropriate treatment and care is not affected by their disclosure. In situations where the patient is unable to give a full history, or when it is felt that the person may be minimising or denying their use, consideration should be given to the fact that alcohol or drugs may be a contributory factor in relation to the current health problem.

A number of standardised alcohol screening instruments exist (Table 11.3) and can be administered quickly as part of routine assessment and history-taking; their use by nurses in the UK has been advocated by the Department of Health (2004). Urine drug screens can aid diagnosis and 'dip sticks' may be helpful in confirming illicit drug use. More detailed analysis can be obtained by sending urine samples to the laboratory for screening, although results will take several days and may therefore not assist in deciding immediate clinical management. The half-life of illicit drugs is vari-

Table 11.3 Standardised alcohol screening tools.

Screening tool	Comments
AUDIT (Alcohol Use Disorders Identification Test)	Developed for use in primary care settings Focuses on identifying patients with hazardous drinking and mild dependence. Scores highly in evaluations of its sensitivity and specificity (Saunders et al., 1993) Its use within the general hospital has been questioned due to the time involved in its administration (Hearne & Connolly, 2002)

CAGE	Acronym stands for:
	    Have you ever felt that you should **C**ut down on your drinking?
	    Have people **A**nnoyed you by criticising your drinking?
	    Have you ever felt **G**uilty about your drinking?
	    Have you ever had a drink first thing in the morning to steady your nerves or get rid of a hangover (**E**ye-opener)?
	Focuses on lifetime alcohol use rather than current drinking
	Quick to administer, but does not ask about frequency of use, levels of consumption or binge drinking
	Advocated for use in primary care and general hospital settings (Armstrong, 1997)
	Alcohol dependence likely if patient answers yes to two or more questions

PAT (Paddington Alcohol Test)	Designed for selective use with adult patients when there is suspicion of excessive alcohol use (Smith et al., 1996). 'Suspicious criteria' would include frequent falls, unexplained blackouts, collapse, assaults, etc. Focuses on amount and frequency of alcohol consumption Designed to be completed in general hospitals (specifically EDs) within 60 seconds

able, for instance amphetamines are detectable in urine up to 48 hours post-administration, cocaine two to three days and methadone seven to nine days (DoH, 1999).

Once it has been identified that substance use is a likely problem, a comprehensive alcohol or drug history needs to be taken, as this will help identify whether the person may benefit from a specialist assessment and referral. The key elements of a detailed alcohol history will include the following:

- amount of alcohol consumed, in units
- rate and pattern of drinking – ask time of first alcoholic drink daily
- history of tolerance to the effects of alcohol
- previous experience of alcohol withdrawal, in particular whether any history of seizures or DT
- signs of any symptoms of dependence or withdrawal
- concomitant use of other substances (either prescribed or illicit drugs)
- any specific behavioural changes associated with alcohol use, e.g. criminal, suicide, sexual, accidents
- potential for suicide, homicide or an accident
- social situation – effects of alcohol on specific issues, e.g. childcare, employment, driving.

In addition to the above, elements of a comprehensive drug-taking history will include:

- substances taken, e.g. amount, duration, frequency. Useful to ask about the daily cost of their habit
- route of use, e.g. oral, smoked, nasal, intravenous
- present or past contact with specialist drug and addiction services
- concomitant use of alcohol
- signs and symptoms of dependence or withdrawal
- social situation – effects that drug misuse has had on this
- presence of behaviours associated with increased risk, e.g. sharing of needles.

Clinical management of alcohol withdrawal

There are often marked variations in the severity of withdrawal symptoms between individual patients, so it is not possible to give exact details of the amount of medication required to treat withdrawal. This should be based on the nature, frequency and severity of the individual patient's symptoms (Box 11.4). When deciding on the amount of medication to be used to manage the features of alcohol withdrawal, attention should be paid to the following:

- The amount of medication required to control symptoms in an individual patient also varies. Factors such as body weight, gender, age and physical

Table 11.4 Suggested medication regimen for the pharmacological withdrawal of alcohol in adults.

Day	Medication	Dose	Frequency
1 and 2	Chlordiazepoxide	20–30 mg	4 × day
3 and 4	Chlordiazepoxide	15 mg	4 × day
5	Chlordiazepoxide	10 mg	4 × day
6	Chlordiazepoxide	10 mg	2 × day
7	Chlordiazepoxide	10 mg	At night

health should be taken in to account when prescribing medication for alcohol withdrawal. Doses of benzodiazepines should be adjusted accordingly for older people. Always refer to the latest edition of the *British National Formulary* before prescribing or administering of benzodiazepines.

■ A reducing regimen of benzodiazepines is usually given over five to ten days (Table 11.4).

■ The precise dose given will depend on the severity of the withdrawal symptoms, the presence of other complications, such as seizures, and how the person has reacted to alcohol withdrawal in the past.

■ Once the benzodiazepine withdrawal regimen is commenced, future dose level will depend on patient response, how well withdrawal symptoms are controlled and the presence, or otherwise, of side effects from treatment, including over sedation or fall in blood pressure.

Individual patients are unlikely to require interventions to manage withdrawal symptoms if:

■ they consume less than 15 units of alcohol daily
■ if binge drinking has lasted less than one week.

Chlordiazepoxide, a long-acting benzodiazepine, is the medication of choice for most patients; it helps prevent seizures and promotes the smooth physiological withdrawal from alcohol. If the patient is to be discharged before the reducing regimen is complete, then caution is required as chlordiazepoxide carries a risk of respiratory depression if the patient resumes alcohol consumption. Stopping abruptly also carries the risk of precipitating withdrawal symptoms. In patients with impaired liver function, chlordiazepoxide metabolism may be affected and consideration should be given to the use of an alternative benzodiazepine, such as lorazepam or oxazepam. If the patient presents with psychotic-type symptoms and marked behavioural disturbance accompanied by perceptual disturbance such as hallucinations, this can be treated by increasing the dose of chlordiazepoxide or adding in a sedative or antipsychotic medication to the treatment plan. The nursing responsibilities for the person who is withdrawing from alcohol are identified in Box 11.5.

> **Box 11.5** The nursing management of acute alcohol withdrawal.
>
> ■ Maintain a non-judgemental attitude – avoid implied or overt criticism
> ■ Use clear, straightforward communication strategies, e.g. avoid complex instructions, maintain eye contact
> ■ Ensure that the person is easily observed
> ■ Monitor vital signs closely – blood pressure, pulse, temperature and respiration
> ■ Ensure adequate hydration – may require intravenous fluids
> ■ Monitor effects and side effects of medication used to manage withdrawal
> ■ Involve the person's family, partner or significant other in the planning and delivery of care if appropriate
> ■ Nurse the person in an area with good lighting and appropriate environmental cues, e.g. clocks that work, calendar, natural light

Clinical management of opiate dependence during hospital admission

As with regular alcohol consumption, admission to hospital will precipitate the sudden cessation of existing opiate use, and although opiate withdrawal is not a life-threatening or particularly hazardous process, it can nevertheless be an extremely distressing experience for the individual. As a result there is a need to minimise the impact of withdrawal and substitute alternatives to illicit opiates. Any clinical management regimen initiated in hospital is not usually continued after discharge unless the person is already being prescribed substitute opiates by a registered practitioner before admission. Taking a proactive approach to the management of the person with opiate dependence while in hospital has the following benefits:

■ Prevention of the experience of unpleasant withdrawal symptoms.
■ Increase in the likelihood of establishing patient concordance with planned treatment and nursing care; if the person is pre-occupied and concerned about withdrawal symptoms, they are less likely to co-operate in medical and nursing treatments.
■ Reduction of the personal, health and social risks associated with the use of illicit drugs, for instance, quantities of opiates used are controlled, the need for the person to engage in antisocial or potentially criminal behaviour is avoided.
■ Provision of opportunities for harm reduction and physical and mental health promotion.

Methadone is the medication of choice for the short-term management of opiate withdrawal within the general hospital. It is an opioid agonist and is used as an opiate substitute. It has a long half-life, ranging from 14 to 72 hours and does not provide the 'rush' that heroin gives. It is itself addictive and

> **Box 11.6** Assessment before commencing methadone in hospital.
>
> **Before prescribing and administration of methadone:**
>
> - Note that it is not to be prescribed for individuals who only use opiates intermittently, i.e. less frequently than daily use, as they will not have developed significant tolerance. Substitute prescribing of methadone to non-opiate dependent drug users can result in overdose
> - Assess accurately the level of drug usage (or methadone prescribing) before the patient was admitted to hospital
> - Clarify with the patient the importance of obtaining accurate information on their pre-admission drug use – seek their co-operation and support
> - Confirm existing use of opiates by urine testing – 'dip sticks'
> - If the person is already receiving methadone in the community, confirm exact details (e.g. amount, frequency, name of prescriber, name of dispenser) by direct contact with the registered prescriber or dispenser. This will also prevent an unauthorised person collecting the prescription while the patient is in hospital
> - Continue the existing dose (if applicable) of methadone during admission
> - Obtain patient's agreement not to attempt to access or use alternative supplies of illicit drugs whilst in hospital
> - Commence methadone prescribing only after confirmation of pre-admission use, or having observed the objective signs of opiate withdrawal (see Table 11.2)
> - Overdose of methadone should be treated with naloxone

can be lethal in overdose, or when taken in combination with other opiates, benzodiazepines or alcohol. Methadone is prescribed as a substitute for heroin to reduce the harm associated with the use of injected illicit drugs. Before commencing methadone it is important to clarify the context and nature of the person's drug use (Box 11.6).

Depending on the reason for admission, some patients who are receiving methadone may require pain relief for the underlying medical or surgical condition. Pain should not be managed by increasing the dose of methadone and, where possible, non-opiate analgesics should be used. However, there may be circumstances where the use of opiate analgesia is indicated, for example, following major surgery, significant trauma involving fractures or soft tissue injuries. It is important to remember that if opiate analgesia is administered in inadequate amounts, or withdrawn too early, it can exacerbate drug-seeking behaviour. See the work of Jage and Bey (2000) for a comprehensive literature review of postoperative analgesia in patients who use illicit drugs. Involving the acute pain services to assist in the development of a specific care plan will be necessary and the plan should outline the future reduction and cessation of the analgesic medication (Welch, 2002). If a patient is being treated with buprenorphine for his drug dependence and is then admitted to hospital and requires pain relief, opiate analgesics should not be used, as these can cause precipitative withdrawal symptoms (DoH, 1999).

Mental health promotion

Excessive alcohol and illicit drug use are best seen as chronic relapsing conditions. While many individuals do bring their alcohol use down to acceptable levels, and those who use illicit drugs are often able to develop a drug-free lifestyle, this is often after repeated attempts to do so, punctuated by periods of relapse and despondency. Admission to hospital with a physical health problem can act as a trigger to behavioural and lifestyle change and can be an ideal opportunity to help the person address the realities of life without alcohol or drugs (Morrison *et al.*, 1997). The adoption of a non-critical and positive manner by the nurse, reinforcing a sense of hope, can assist in helping the person consider whether he or she is ready to address the issue of making changes in their current lifestyle.

General nurses often feel anxious regarding their knowledge and ability to deal with alcohol and drug problems (Lockart, 1997). There may also be negative attitudes towards this group, seeing them as 'time wasters', or as unable to change their behaviour (Herring & Thom, 1999). As a result, staff need to receive specific training as a way of increasing their confidence and skills in this area. Negative beliefs and attitudes about patients with these problems can also be addressed through training, clinical supervision and appropriate management support, for example, the development of clinical guidelines and relevant policies.

The Royal College of Physicians (2001) describe the need for general hospital staff to move beyond just treating the presenting alcohol-related problem or physical illness, to a position where they are able to help the person focus on the underlying alcohol problem, including health promotion activity. A number of theoretical perspectives exist that help in our understanding of the factors impacting upon personal change. These include Prochaska and Di Clemente's 'Stages of change' model (1982) and the brief intervention approach advocated by Miller and Sanchez (1993). Both provide a framework by which the health professional can address the issue of change, motivation and personal responsibility with the person concerned. Whatever model is adopted, it is important to remember that not every patient will recognise the need to change, or be ready and willing to address the fact that they need to change. For example, this can become apparent after providing information about the health risks of excessive alcohol, when the provision of information alone is usually not adequate to ensure that the person discontinues their harmful alcohol use. Nursing staff need to be sensitive to this and recognise that it may take a number of opportunities and numerous attempts before the individual is personally ready to address the need to change their lifestyle and behaviour.

Table 11.5 The FRAMES approach to brief intervention (adapted from Miller & Sanchez, 1993).

Feedback	Feedback by the nurse on their assessment of the problem
Responsibility	Advise the patient that drinking is their responsibility
Advice	Give clear advice, both written and verbal, as to the reasons why there is a need to stop drinking
Menu	Help the patient to identify a range ('menu') of options or choices regarding their drinking behaviour
Empathy	Be empathic, warm, understanding and encouraging about the person's ability to change
Self-efficiency	Encourage and reinforce the person's ability to achieve change by being self-reliant, e.g. avoid blaming others for their problems or failure to achieve an alcohol-free lifestyle

Adopting a brief intervention focus, that acknowledges that the time and opportunities for health promotion and implementing behavioural change may be limited, has been shown to help reduce harmful substance use. Brief interventions are those aimed at promoting moderation or harm-free drinking and involve:

- Assessment and identification
- Advice
- Counselling with education
- Promotion of self-help.

The common elements of brief intervention have been summarised by the acronym FRAMES (see Table 11.5), which provides a framework that the non-specialist can use to address the need for personal change.

In order to ensure that the chances of change are maximised, and that individual patients receive the appropriate level of specialist help when discharged from hospital, nursing teams need to develop contacts and links with local non-statutory and specialist drug services. Much informal support, counselling, advice and treatment is provided by non-statutory agencies such as Alcoholics Anonymous (AA) and Narcotics Anonymous (NA), so it is necessary to know the local contacts and means of access or referral. The mental health liaison team can provide a link between hospital-based services and specialist drug, alcohol and addictions services (see Chapter 6).

Conclusions

The problems of excessive alcohol and illicit drug use are common, and the consequences of each are seen frequently by clinicians working in the general hospital. The screening and assessment of these problems is generally poor, although there is increasing recognition of the potentially important role that all nurses have in identification and treatment of the health and social consequences arising from the use of these substances. The undesirable effects of alcohol in particular are the cause of much concern and need to become the focus for all health care staff working within the general hospital. The use of standardised screening instruments has been shown to be effective in identifying those individuals who can benefit from targeted health promotion and supportive interventions. This chapter has also outlined the safe and effective care of those patients requiring specific interventions when experiencing acute alcohol or opiate withdrawal as a means of ensuring the delivery of patient-focused nursing.

References

Agarwal, D.P. (2002) Review: cardioprotective effects of light-moderate consumption of alcohol: a review of putative mechanisms. *Alcohol and Alcoholism*, 37 (5): 409–415.

Allen, J., Litters, R.Z. & Lee, A. (1998) What you need to know: detecting alcohol problems in general medical practice. *Singapore Medical Journal*, 39: 38–41.

Armstrong, E. (1997) *The Primary Mental Health Care Toolkit*. London: Royal College of General Practitioners.

Ashworth, M. & Gerada, C. (1997) ABC of mental health: Addiction and dependence – II: alcohol. *British Medical Journal*, 315: 358–360.

Crowe, A.V., Howse M. & Bell G.M. (2000) Substance abuse and the kidney. *Quarterly Journal of Medicine*, 93: 47–152.

Department of Health (1995) *Interdepartmental Working Group: sensible drinking*. London: HMSO.

Department of Health (1999) *Drug Misuse and Dependence – guidelines on clinical management*. London: HMSO.

Department of Health (2004) Detecting alcohol abuse earlier. *The CNO Bulletin*, December 2004/January 2005: 8.

Hearne, R. & Connolly, A. (2002) Alcohol abuse: prevalence and detection in a general hospital. *Journal of the Royal Society of Medicine*, 95: 84–87.

Herring, R. & Thom, B. (1999) 'Resisting the gaze'? Nurses' perception of the role of Accident and Emergency department in responding to alcohol-related attendances. *Critical Public Health*, 9 (2): 135–148.

Jage, B. & Bey, T. (2000) Postoperative analgesia in patients with substance use disorders: Part 1. *International Journal of Acute Pain Management*, 3: 40–155.

Kushner, S.F. (1991) Substance abuse and neurological disorders. In: M.S. Gold & A. Slaby (eds) *Dual Diagnosis in Substance Abuse*, pp. 75–103. New York: Marcel Dekker.

Lockhart, T. (1997) Problem drinkers in accident and emergency: health promotion initiatives. *Accident and Emergency*, 5: 16–21.

Miller, W.R. & Sanchez, V.C. (1993) Motivating young adults for treatment and lifestyle changes. In: G. Howard (ed.) *Issues in Alcohol Use and Misuse in Young Adults*. Notre Dame: University of Notre Dame Press.

Morrison, A., Elliott, L. & Gruer, L. (1997) Injecting-related harm and treatment seeking behaviour among injecting drug users. *Addiction*, 92 (10): 1349–1352.

Pomeroy, C. (2002) Alcohol and drug abuse. In: C. Pomeroy (ed.) *Medical Complications of Psychiatric Illness*, pp. 175–203. Washington: American Psychiatric Publishing Inc.

Prochaska, J.Q. & Di Clemente, C.C. (1982) Transtheoretical therapy: towards a more integrative model of change. *Psychotherapy: Theory, Research and Practice*, 19: 276–288.

Royal College of Physicians (2001) *Alcohol: can the NHS afford it?* London: Royal College of Physicians.

Royal College of Physicians, Royal College of Psychiatrists and Royal College of General Practitioners (1995) *Alcohol and the Heart in Perspective: sensible limits reaffirmed*. London: RCP/RCPsych/RCGP.

Saunders, J.B., Aasland, O.G. & Bobor, T.F. (1993) Development of the Alcohol Use Disorders Identification Test (AUDIT): W.H.O. collaborative project on early detection of persons with harmful alcohol consumption, part II. *Addiction*, 88: 791–804.

Smith, S.G.T., Touquet, R. & Wright, S. (1996) Detection of alcohol misusing patients in accident and emergency departments: the Paddington Alcohol Test. *Journal of Accident and Emergency Medicine*, 13: 308–312.

UK Alcohol Forum (2001) *Guidelines For the Management of Alcohol Problems in Primary Care and General Psychiatry*, 2nd edn. High Wycombe: Tangent Medical Education.

Waller, S., Thom, B. & Harris, S. (1998) Perception of alcohol related attendances in A and E departments in England: a national survey. *Alcohol and Alcoholism*, 33 (4): 354–361.

Welch, S. (2002) Management of substance misuse problems in the general hospital. *Clinical Medicine*, 2 (6): 513–515.

World Health Organization (1992) *International Classification of Impairments, Disabilities and Handicaps*. Geneva: WHO.

World Health Organization (2003) *International Classification of Diseases and Related Health Problems 10*. Geneva: WHO.

Chapter 12
Caring for Older People with Mental Health Problems

Chapter aims

> ### This chapter will:
>
> - identify the common mental health problems experienced by older people within the general hospital
> - discuss the impact of ageism on the perception of mental health and illness
> - outline the principles of an holistic nursing assessment
> - describe the presentation, clinical management and nursing care required for the person suffering from dementia and confusion.

Introduction

The provision of effective care for individuals with mental health problems in acute hospitals, intermediate care units and community hospitals is a complex activity, requiring the commitment of a range of health and social care professionals. The provision of psychological and emotional care is often seen as the remit of mental health specialists, rather than of the general nurse. Older people have a number of specific needs in relation to the provision of mental health care, and this applies specifically to the general hospital, where there are high rates of psychiatric morbidity (Bowler *et al.*, 1994). Despite this, there is evidence that older people with mental health problems are often excluded from mainstream health care (Sherratt & Younger-Ross, 2004), and there is often poor collaboration between acute care and mental health services.

The *National Service Framework for Older People* (Department of Health (DoH), 2001a), challenges nurses to deliver care that is person-centred and addresses the person's mental health needs. However, this can only be delivered if all those involved in the process acknowledge the need to work

Table 12.1 Prevalence of psychiatric illness in older people.

	General population	General hospital
Depression	10%	65%
Acute confusion (delirium)	6%	60%
Anxiety disorders	5%	10%
Psychotic disorders	1%	9%
Dementia	5%	25%

RCN, 1997; Woods, 1999; Burns *et al.*, 2002

together, starting with the planning and commissioning of services, and underpinned by the ability of practitioners to provide safe and effective patient-focused care.

Prevalence of mental health problems

There has been a rise of 9% in the UK population who are over 65 since 1900; predictions are that the older adult population will exceed 25% by 2041 (Office of Population Censuses Surveys, 1987). Psychiatric illness is high in this group, but many problems go undetected and untreated. The prevalence of psychiatric morbidity in older people within the general hospital is higher than the general population (Burns *et al.*, 2002), although it is difficult to be precise about rates due to the wide variation of diagnostic criteria used in various population studies (Table 12.1).

Despite high prevalence rates, evidence exists as to the lack of co-ordinated care for older people when in hospital, with national reports identifying significant gaps in the provision of mental health care (Audit Commission, 2000; Holmes *et al.*, 2002). The reasons for this are multi-factorial, but many are linked to the dualistic notions of health discussed in Chapters 2 and 3. The impact of ageism, whereby older people are often viewed as a 'burden', or as being problematic and unpopular, also contributes to the perception that this group of individuals is more difficult to look after and less rewarding to care for.

The impact of ageism

There is often a view that illness and infirmity are an inevitable result of ageing, as well as a belief that little can be done for a person once they reach a certain age; these views are more likely to be applied to older people who have mental health problems (Page *et al.*, 2003). Stereotypical images may be reinforced by media representations, the use of pejorative language, and the general lack of value ascribed to older people in society.

Such views have a negative impact on the provision of health care generally and nursing care in particular (DoH, 2001a,b). Older people with mental health problems are likely to have difficulty in accessing care due to the discrimination experienced as a result of their age, and the fact that they are suffering from problems that are often seen as less amenable to treatment than those resulting from a physical illness (Hunt, 1993). Nurses working in general hospitals cite blurring of role boundaries, lack of time, communication difficulties and lack of skill and knowledge as the main difficulties associated with providing effective care for older adults with mental health needs (Bridges, 2001).

Many of these 'difficulties' are linked to the practitioner's previous experience and preconceptions about how the person will behave. Underlying beliefs may result in the person being cared for in a way that lacks attention to individual need, is negative and views them as burdensome (Norman, 1997). Hospital care for older people is seen by some as sub-standard and there continue to be major challenges in improving the care and treatment for patients with mental health needs (Nazarko, 2004). However, despite such problems, there are examples where non-mental health staff have responded to this aspect of nursing in a positive and proactive way (Wightman, 2001; Hickling, 2004).

Assessment

Accurate assessment is essential in order that care can be delivered in a patient-focused way. Many of the difficulties cited by nursing staff when caring for people with mental health problems can be traced back to inadequate attention to initial assessment and history taking, compounded by professionals who feel inadequate about their ability to accurately identify psychological morbidity (Tucker *et al.*, 2001).

The *National Service Framework for Older People* (DoH, 2001a) tasks all health and social care services with delivering care that is person-centred, in order to avoid inappropriate assessments, duplication, repetition and poor inter-service communication. Alongside this, the Single Assessment Process (SAP) has been developed to ensure that professionals adopt a holistic view of the patient and their health and social care needs. It enables the physical, psychological and social domains of care to be addressed within a single assessment framework (DoH, 2004). There is an expectation that all health and social care agencies will use the SAP (Box 12.1) as the process whereby the older person's health and social needs are assessed and communicated between the various organisations involved. Mental health needs make up a significant component of this framework. The SAP provides a template for patient and carer assessment, along with mechanisms for ensuring that relevant information is shared between health and social care agencies. Hospital-based assessments should form a key component of the SAP (Royal College of Nursing, 2004).

> **Box 12.1** The Single Assessment Process (DoH, 2004).
>
> Requires detailed assessment of the following aspects of the person's health and social care:
>
> - User's perspective of their needs and priorities
> - Nutrition
> - Activities of daily living
> - Pain
> - Oral health
> - Tissue viability
> - Mobility and balance
> - Falls
> - Communication, visual and hearing disability
> - Cognitive impairment/memory
> - General mental health
> - Depression/anxiety/mood
> - Relationships
> - Impact of caring on family carers
> - Housing

Effective nursing assessment provides the basis for the planning and delivery of holistic care, as well as helping to identify the need for further investigations and treatment. It is dependent upon the nurse's skills of observation, interviewing and examination. A comprehensive assessment will place equal emphasis upon mental and physical health, although traditionally much documentation has focused on physical health care needs, as opposed to an assessment that addresses all the elements that go to make up the older person (Wills & Ford, 2001). Non-psychiatric staff should be able to undertake a baseline mental health assessment as part of an overall nursing assessment. Guidelines for completing this have been developed by the Royal College of Nursing (1997) and consist of the following core elements:

- Mood, cognitive abilities and behaviour. Exploration of how the person is feeling currently; evidence of depression, elation, anxiety or frustration
- The need to develop an understanding of the person's social and health history, including details of how they function in their usual surroundings. Chronology and timescales relating to the development of the person's health problems.
- Effective assessment requires the nurse to:
  - possess effective interpersonal skills and the ability to form therapeutic relationships
  - develop adequate self-awareness, acknowledging the impact of personal beliefs and behaviours, role boundaries and the need for appropriate levels of education and clinical supervision

Box 12.2 Baseline mental health assessment information.

Presenting history. What were the precipitants to this problem? Consider the likely causes of the person's current distress, e.g. pain and discomfort, side effects of medication, recent anaesthesia, stress, underlying medical illness, alcohol withdrawal, etc.

Utilising observation and questioning techniques, note the following:

- *General behaviour and attitude.* Include details of amount of eye contact, facial expression and interaction with others
- *Speech.* Note whether slow, rapid, hesitant, loud, comprehensible, whether content is appropriate to situation; whenever possible document the person's own words and phrases
- *Cognitive functioning.* Whether the person understands what is happening and why they are here; concentration and attention, memory and recall; whether orientated to time, place and person; thoughts, preoccupations; any evidence of delusions or hallucinations
- *Current mood.* Note whether tense, depressed, anxious, excited, elated, hostile; whether mood is consistent or liable to sudden changes

   □ identify the most appropriate screening tools to support effective assessment

   □ pay attention to the person's strengths as well as their deficits and problems.

A template for undertaking such an assessment can be developed and incorporated into standard nursing documentation (Box 12.2). This provides a measure against which to judge changes in the patient's mental state.

When a mental health problem is suspected, or the person is considered at risk of developing one, the use of screening instruments can be helpful in quantifying the problem (Table 12.2). Most screening instruments require

Table 12.2 Screening tools that may be used with older people.

Screening tool	Comments
Abbreviated Mental Test (AMT)	A 10-item screening tool that tests aspects of memory and orientation
Geriatric Depression Scale (GDS)	Available in a 15-item and 30-item version. Self-report questionnaire, using yes/no responses
Mini-Mental State Examination (MMSE)	An 11-item screening tool. Assesses aspects of memory, orientation, attention, language and registration
Hospital Anxiety and Depression Scale (HADS)	A 14-item self-report questionnaire designed to screen for anxiety and depression in general hospital patients

those administering them to have received further training in their use, in particular when deciding on the significance, or otherwise, of the results. When such results suggest a clinical problem, then the patient is likely to require further specialist assessment. Such screening tools bring a 'quasi-scientific approach' to the assessment of a person's mental state, but they should be seen as an adjunct to assessment and not be used as diagnostic tools, or to place the person into a particular patient group or diagnostic category (Royal College of Nursing, 1997).

Dementia

Dementia is a common problem within the general hospital, with significantly higher rates than in community settings. Dementia is not a diagnosis, rather it is a cluster of symptoms that provide a label for a range of specific behavioural, psychological and physical deficits. Various sub-types exist, including vascular dementia, Alzheimer's disease, Lewy body dementia, alcoholic dementia and Creutzfeldt–Jakob disease (Table 12.3).

Dementia affects over 700 000 people (Page et al., 2003), and the incidence increases with age. Many symptoms and problems will follow an increasingly chronic course, and are likely to include a number of physical health problems. Despite the frequency with which dementia is seen, many nurses respond negatively and fail to address patient need effectively (Page & Burgess, 2003).

The various types of dementia all have common symptoms, but a diagnosis can only be confirmed following specialist assessment, computed tomography (CT) and brain scanning. Arriving at a diagnosis may be difficult and is largely a process of exclusion. Accurate history and thorough assessment is vital, particularly as the features are often similar to those seen in other forms of confusion, such as delirium (Table 12.4). Staff may then assume that the person is suffering from dementia, when in fact their confusion is due to an underlying organic cause. This can lead to mismanaging ongoing care needs, and may even result in inappropriate placement in residential and nursing care (Dewing, 2001a).

The onset of dementia is generally insidious, often not coming to the attention of health staff until the person attends for physical complaints or symptoms. A precipitant to sudden deterioration in mental and social functioning can be a life event that disrupts the person's usual routine, such as a bereavement or admission to hospital for treatment of a physical health problem. The person may present as more confused, anxious or unable to cope. Features of dementia affect all aspects of the individual's emotional, physical, social and interpersonal wellbeing (Table 12.5). Psychiatric symptoms, such as depression and hallucinations, may also be present. Nursing care needs to address both physical and psychological problems. If dementia is suspected, referral for further specialist assessment will be required.

Table 12.3 The various types of dementia and their causes.

Form of dementia	Notes
Alzheimer's disease	Most common form of dementia – accounts for approximately 50% of cases Cause unknown Thought to occur as a result of development of plaques within the temporal and parietal lobes, leading to disruption of the neurotransmitter system
Vascular dementia	Accounts for approximately 20% of cases Linked to development of arteriosclerosis in the brain; caused when small clots are carried to the cortical areas and lead to patches of ischaemia Untreated hypertension is a risk factor
Lewy body dementia	Lewy bodies are pink-staining structures found in the cytoplasm of neurones Dementia-like symptoms caused by the profusion of Lewy bodies in the brain stem and cortical areas Causes significant impairment of parietal lobe functioning, differs from the other forms of dementia in that marked memory loss is less common Common symptoms include visual and auditory hallucinations, fluctuating between confusion and lucidity, and unexplained falls Patients with Lewy body dementia should not be given antipsychotic medication, as these cause rapid onset extrapyramidal symptoms (see Chapter 10)
Creutzfeldt–Jakob disease	Caused by infective proteins known as prions Rapid onset, with a poor prognosis Can affect any age group
Alcoholic dementia	Develops as a result of long-term excessive alcohol consumption, also known as Korsakoff's syndrome Caused by a lack of vitamin B complex, most notably thiamine Patient presents with impaired memory, confabulation (making up stories to explain things) and disorientation to time and place Vitamin replacement and cessation of drinking will lead to improvement, if given early enough

There are a number of newer pharmacological treatments for dementia using medications called anticholinesterases. These act by preventing the breakdown of acetylcholine, the neurotransmitter that is deficient in patients with Alzheimer's disease. Other psychotropic medications may be prescribed to treat specific cognitive or behavioural symptoms, although all should be

Table 12.4 Differentiation between dementia and delirium.

	Dementia	**Delirium – acute confusion**
Onset	Slow – months and years	Rapid – hours or days
Presentation	Alert, but disorientated Can present as calm and co-operative	Fluctuating consciousness Disorientated to time, place, person Agitated and difficult to reassure
Speech	Maintains ability to have conversation	Bizarre ideas and conversation
Perception	Hallucinations in 30% of cases, otherwise no abnormality	Visual hallucinations common
Insight	Fluctuating – in early stages person presents with periods of lucidity and awareness of their cognitive decline	Minimal insight, difficult to reason with, often not reassured by explanation
Depressive symptoms	Common	Uncommon, likely to present as anxious and agitated

used judiciously, and rarely as a first-line treatment option (Table 12.6). Antipsychotic medication should not be used in patients without psychotic symptoms. In some patients they may be poorly tolerated and can make symptoms worse (Burns *et al.*, 2002).

Nursing interventions

Providing care within an acute setting poses significant challenges. The impact of an unfamiliar environment, strange tasks and rituals, and the individual's communication difficulties are all likely to increase stress and hinder the person's ability to comply with staff expectations. It is easy for staff to adopt a mechanistic approach, paying limited attention to the person's individual needs, so that the experience of being in hospital detracts from recovery. A number of factors will impact on the patient's ability to adjust, and these need to be considered when planning and delivering nursing care (Pritchard & Dewing, 2001). Examples include:

- unfamiliar ward routines and rituals
- the way in which staff approach the patient
- feeling unwell and bewildered
- trying to cope with change when it is unclear what that change is and why it is occurring
- being isolated and treated differently from other patients on the ward.

Table 12.5 The features of dementia.

Aspect of the person	Notes
Memory impairment	Often noticed first by relatives or friends May be so gradual that it is difficult to date the onset Short-term memory is affected first – longer-term recall may remain intact for a long time Often begins with failure to remember names, appointments, etc.; eventually leads to profound forgetfulness, such as forgetting the way on a familiar journey, confusion over previously mastered tasks in the home
Personality changes	Intellectual changes and decrease in social awareness May become obsessive or develop over-valued ideas, often relating to physical health May display irritability, excessive stubbornness, lack of awareness for the feelings of others
Thinking	Becomes slowed and restrictive Difficulty in coping with new ideas; thinking becomes 'concrete' Reduced concentration, easily tired by having to think Ability to think and reason is lost In later stages, poverty of thought is demonstrated by slowed speech, which may eventually become a series of incomprehensible words or phrases
Behaviour	Social withdrawal 20% will display aggression 25% will 'wander' 40% will experience some form of incontinence 5% will display sexual disinhibition
Psychiatric symptoms	Between 30% and 50% will present with delusions, paranoid ideas, visual and auditory hallucinations, and misidentification
Physical	Loss of energy In later stages, person is likely to experience problems with eating and diet, washing, dressing, personal hygiene, mobility, expressing sexuality
Communication	Communication may occur in ways considered disruptive or 'unacceptable' by staff, and may include shouting, wandering and hitting out Communication difficulties are often the result of frustration at not being able to make needs and feelings understood Aphasia – may be expressive (unable to communicate verbally), or receptive (unable to process and understand verbal communications of others) Apraxia – increasing difficulty in undertaking skilled movements Agnosia – difficulty in understanding and interpreting familiar objects

Dewing, 2001a; Burns *et al.*, 2002; Bush, 2003

Table 12.6 Psychotropic medication that may be prescribed during the treatment of dementia.

Medication group	Examples	Notes
Anticholinesterases	Donepezil Rivastigmine Galantamine Memantine	For use in patients with Alzheimer's disease Must be prescribed by a psychiatrist and management reviewed by mental health specialists (NICE, 2001) Improve general cognitive functioning and memory Most common side effects are gastrointestinal, e.g. nausea
Antipsychotics	Haloperidol Olanzapine	Used to manage markedly disturbed or agitated behaviour Should not be used in patients with Lewy body dementia Should only be used as a last-line treatment Has the potential to exacerbate symptoms of behavioural disturbance Risperidone should be prescribed with caution in patients with dementia, as it increases the risk of stroke (CSM, 2004)
Benzodiazepines	Diazepam Lorazepam Chlordiazepoxide	Can be used to produce a short-term calming effect Can cause over-sedation and respiratory depression For short-term use only, i.e. no longer than one week's continuous use

It is necessary to appreciate that behaviour which is viewed as difficult or problematic by staff is likely to be the only way in which the individual has to communicate. In order to develop a patient-focused agenda, a number of factors need to be incorporated into the planning and delivery of care (Table 12.7).

The use of restraint and the routine administration of psychotropic medication as a means of managing challenging behaviour is almost always unjustified and rarely addresses the person's underlying needs. Alternative interventions (Watson, 2002) should be considered, including:

- Assessment and treatment of underlying physical illness
- Thorough assessment of mental state and treatment of underlying mental illness, e.g. depression
- Alleviation of pain and discomfort
- Modification of the environment
- Provision of space and emotional security
- Review of the use of previously prescribed medication.

Table 12.7 Factors necessary for effective care of the person with dementia.

Domain of care	Nursing interventions
Communication	Avoid approaching from behind – always approach from the front Address person by their preferred name – use his or her name frequently Use short, straightforward language – enunciate clearly When asking questions, pose them one at a time Focus on how the person is feeling, rather than asking what he or she thinks, e.g. 'How does it feel to be wearing this shirt?' 'How do you feel now that you have got out of bed?' Allow enough time for the person to respond – be aware that your need to 'get things done' is likely to be the opposite of the individual's need for time and patience Be prepared to repeat requests or questions Avoid phrases such as, 'Walk over here'. Use specific terms such as, 'Please walk over to the table' Negative phrases are likely to reinforce the person's sense of failure and helplessness, so use positive statements, avoiding commands such as 'Don't' and 'No' Ensure you are able to give the person your undivided attention – see each activity as an opportunity to engage and promote a sense of well-being and emotional security. Avoid viewing contacts as a series of tasks, focus on using activity as a way of attending to the person's emotional needs
Environment	Try to ensure consistency of contact – identify named nurses to plan and provide care, rather than assign temporary staff Avoid changes to bed space and the person's immediate environment Do not isolate the person in a side room – lack of visual and verbal contact is likely to increase isolation, possibly leading to more frequent displays of negative communication Ensure adequate lighting and easily readable signs Make conscious and realistic attempts to help the person maintain a daily routine Encourage the person's partner to bring in familiar objects that can act as visual reminders
Effective use of self	Reflect on your approach to the person – what is your agenda (e.g. 'To get all the washes done')? Such a task-focus will detract from providing patient-orientated care. Your underlying agenda is also communicated in other ways, such as tone of voice, body posture and the way in which you approach the person Identify the person's needs, rather than what you want to achieve Pay attention to non-verbal communication, e.g. how irritated or frustrated do you feel? Such cues are likely to make the person agitated and reinforce a negative pattern of interpersonal communication
Psychological care	Look for clues as to what the person's behaviour may mean – what is he or she trying to tell you? Start your interactions with the intention of helping the person to have their needs met, as opposed to focusing on addressing your professional needs

Table 12.7 (Cont'd)

Domain of care	Nursing interventions
Carer's needs	Enlist the help and support of carers with the provision of everyday care, having first ascertained what level of involvement the carer is comfortable with and realistically able to provide
	Use formal and informal means of assessing carer's needs. Help them to access appropriate help, support and care that will enable them to address their physical and mental health needs
	Engage the person's carer as an equal partner – you may have professional expertise, but the carer is likely to know the person to a much greater degree than you ever will
	Adopt a non-judgemental approach regarding the degree of involvement the carer is willing to offer. Not every carer will have the physical and emotional resources required to support their relative through the various stages of dementia

Based on Dewing, 2001a; 2003.

Acute confusion (delirium)

Delirium is a problem affecting approximately 20% of patients in general wards, with the incidence rising to 60% for those with critical illnesses (Hughes, 2001). Despite such prevalence, there is evidence that it is poorly understood and inadequately treated. Strictly speaking, delirium is not a mental illness, although the patient presents with a range of symptoms that may mimic psychiatric illness (Table 12.8). Delirium is associated with increased mortality, increased nursing observation, failed rehabilitation and delayed hospital discharge. Delirium is a symptom, not a diagnosis, and frequently indicates a severe but treatable underlying illness. The risk factors for the development of delirium are:

- Individuals over 80 years of age
- Extremely physically frail
- Multiple medical problems
- Infections, particularly chest and urinary tract
- Polypharmacy
- Sensory impairment
- Metabolic disturbance
- Long-bone fractures
- General anaesthesia.

Onset is always abrupt, usually within hours or days. Nearly all cases are reversible when the underlying cause is treated. However, there are occasions when staff fail to recognise delirium, leading to delays in appropriate treatment and an overall worsening of the underlying condition (Schofield & Dewing, 2001). Obtaining an accurate history from the patient, their partner or another family member can speed diagnosis. The Confusion Assessment

Table 12.8 Characteristic features of delirium.

Feature	Notes
Disorientation	Frequently disorientated to time, place and person
Impaired concentration and attention	Unable to focus or follow conversation
Altered cognitive state	May appear to be looking around anxiously; appears frightened, difficult for staff to provide reassurance
Altered perception	Misinterpretation of external stimuli – may experience visual hallucinations
Memory	Poor short- and long-term recall
Impaired ability to communicate	Confused, prone to wander, apparently 'odd' conversations that appear meaningless to others. May appear unco-operative
Disturbed sleep–wake cycle	Often manifests as insomnia and increased levels of nocturnal agitation – may start as early as late afternoon/early evening
Increased psychomotor activity	May show signs of irritability and apparent aggression

Method (CAM) has been developed as a specific nursing assessment tool aimed at identifying those suffering from delirium (Inouye *et al.*, 1990). The CAM identifies four core features of delirium, at least three of which need to be present in order to establish its presence (Box 12.3).

Because of the often overt displays of behavioural distress associated with delirium, it can be tempting to consider that these problems are 'psychiatric' in origin. This perspective only serves to reinforce the erroneous belief that there is little that can be done for the person. However, it is important to recognise that sensitive, patient-focused nursing can positively influence both the degree of distress experienced and the duration of the illness. In this way, nurses are less likely to resort to the overuse of strategies such as the administration of psychotropic medication as a means of responding to the person's confused state (Dewing, 2001b). It is essential to ensure that the relevant investigations and treatments for the underlying cause are implemented (Box 12.4).

The nursing contribution to caring for a person experiencing acute confusion is a major strand of the treatment and care while in hospital. A number of preventive measures can be taken as a strategy for reducing the impact and duration of confused and disorientated behaviours. Such measures include:

- Communication aimed at orientating the person to the environment.
- Strategies to make the environment more familiar, such as use of signs and personal possessions, wall clocks that function and display the correct time, written information sheets.
- Continuity of staff.
- Involvement of partner, family, friends.
- Minimising the impact of excessive noise, non-essential visits from non-ward based staff; promotion of adequate sleep by avoiding non-essential nursing interventions during the night.

Box 12.3 The Confusion Assessment Method.

Feature 1: Acute onset and fluctuating course

This feature is confirmed by discussion with a family member/significant other, or a member of staff. It is demonstrated by positive responses to the following questions:

- Is there evidence of an acute change in mental status from the patient's baseline?
- Did the abnormal behaviour fluctuate during the day – i.e. did it tend to come and go, or increase or decrease in severity?

Feature 2: Inattention

Demonstrated by a positive response to the following question:

- Did the patient have difficulty in focusing attention, e.g. being easily distractible, or have difficulty keeping track of what was being said?

Feature 3: Disorganised thinking

Demonstrated by a positive response to the following question:

- Was the patient's thinking disorganised or incoherent, such as rambling or irrelevant speech, unclear or illogical flow of ideas, or unpredictable switching from subject to subject?

Feature 4: Altered level of consciousness

Demonstrated by the patient presenting with any one of the following:

- Vigilance (hyperalert)
- Lethargy (drowsy, but easily aroused)
- Stupor (difficult to arouse)
- Coma (unrousable)

A diagnosis of delirium by CAM requires the presence of features 1 & 2 and either 3 or 4.

(Cited in Schofield & Dewing, 2001). Reproduced with permission of the RCN Publishing Company.

> **Box 12.4** An overview of the assessment and clinical management of delirium.
>
> - Identify and treat the underlying cause – return to baseline or pre-morbid state can take up to three weeks
> - Ensure all appropriate laboratory tests and investigations are completed, e.g. full blood count, viscosity, urea and electrolytes, blood glucose, liver function, thyroid function, urine screen, chest X-ray
> - Ensure complete physical examination has taken place, including neurological and rectal
> - Rule out acute alcohol withdrawal – initiate alcohol withdrawal regimen if necessary (see Chapter 11).
> - Always assume an underlying organic cause, particularly in the absence of a pre-existing history of cognitive impairment
> - Ensure adequate hydration and dietary intake
> - Use clear, straightforward communication strategies, e.g. short sentences, avoid use of jargon and expressions that may be taken literally, maintain eye contact, make positive statements rather than reinforcing the patient's failure or non-co-operation
> - Orientate the person to his/her environment; provide reassurance in the form of explanation – this may need to be repeated frequently

Conclusions

There are high rates of psychiatric morbidity within the general hospital and other physical care settings. Nurses caring for people with a physical illness have an important part to play in the assessment, treatment and ongoing management of mental health problems. During the patient's journey, it is often at this point that mental health difficulties are either missed or inadequately treated and managed. It is therefore vital that nursing staff possess the necessary knowledge, skills and attitudes to address these problems. This chapter has identified the importance of adopting a holistic approach to the assessment and nursing care for such patients, while identifying the impact that stereotypical beliefs and negative attitudes can have upon the delivery of this vital area of care.

References

Audit Commission (2000) *Forget Me Not*. London: Audit Commission.

Bowler, C., Boyle, A. & Branford, M. (1994) Detection of psychiatric disorders in elderly medical inpatients. *Age and Ageing*, 23 (4): 307–311.

Bridges, J. (2001) Improving rehabilitation care. *Nursing Times*, 97 (4): 37–38.

Burns, A., Purandare, N. & Craig, S. (2002) *Mental Health in Older People in Practice*. London: The Royal Society of Medicine Press.

Bush, T. (2003) Communicating with patients who have dementia. *Nursing Times*, 99 (48): 42–45.

Committee on the Safety of Medicines (2004) *New Advice Issued on Risperidone and Olanzapine: 2004/0095*. London: DoH.

Department of Health (2001a) *National Service Framework for Older People*. London: DoH.

Department of Health (2001b) *Caring for Older People: Integrating Knowledge, Practice and Values*. London: DoH.

Department of Health (2004) *Single Assessment Process for Older People – April 2004 Milestone*. London: DoH.

Dewing, J. (2001a) Care for people with a dementia in acute hospital settings. *Nursing Older People*, 13 (3): 18–20.

Dewing, J. (2001b) The nursing contribution to the care of older people with delirium in acute care settings. *Nursing Older People*, 13 (1): 21–25.

Dewing, J. (2003) Rehabilitation for older people with dementia. *Nursing Standard*, 18 (6): 42–48.

Hickling, K. (2004) Improving the awareness of depression in older people. *Nursing Times*, 100 (27): 47.

Holmes, J., Bentley, K. & Cameron, I. (2002) *Between Two Stools: psychiatric services for older people in general hospitals*. Leeds: University of Leeds.

Hughes, A. (2001) Recognising the causes of delirium in older people. *Nursing Times*, 97 (33): 32–33.

Hunt, E. (1993) On avoiding 'psych' patients. *Journal of Emergency Nursing*, 19 (5): 375–376.

Inouye, S., Van Dyck, C.H. & Alessi, C.A. (1990) Clarifying confusion: The Confusion Assessment Method: A new method for the detection of delirium. *Annals of Internal Medicine*, 3 (12): 941–948.

National Institute for Clinical Excellence (2001) *Guidance on the Use of Donepezil, Rivastigmine and Galantamine for the Treatment of Alzheimer's Disease*. London: NICE.

Nazarko, L. (2004) How clinical governance can enhance care for older people. *Nursing Times*, 100 (11): 42–45.

Norman, I. (1997) Supporting paid carers. In: I.J. Norman & S.J. Redfern (eds). *Mental Health Care for Elderly People*. Edinburgh: Churchill Livingstone.

Office of Population Censuses and Surveys (1987) *Population Projections 1985–2025*. London: HMSO.

Page, S. & Burgess, L. (2003) Educating nursing staff involved in the provision of dementia care. *Nursing Times*, 99 (46): 34–37.

Page, S., Hardman, P. & Burgess, L. (2003) Changing attitudes in dementia care and the role of nurses. *Nursing Times*, 99 (38): 18–19.

Pritchard, E. & Dewing, J. (2001) Older people with dementia in acute settings. *Nursing Older People*, 12 (10): 21–25.

Royal College of Nursing (1997) *Guidelines for Assessing Mental Health Needs in Old Age*. London: RCN.

Royal College of Nursing (2004) *Nursing Assessment and Older People*. London: RCN.

Schofield, I. & Dewing, J. (2001) The nursing contribution to the care of older people with a delirium in acute care settings. *Nursing Older People*, 13 (1): 21–25.

Sherratt, C. & Younger-Ross, S. (2004) Out of sight out of mind. *Community Care*, 29 April–5 May: 40–41.

Tucker, S., Darley, J. & Cullum, S. (2001) How to detect and manage depression in older people. *Nursing Times*, 97 (45): 36–37.

Watson, R. (2002) Assessing the need for restraint in older people. *Nursing Older People*, 14 (4): 31–32.

Wightman, S. (2001) Dementia care. *Nursing Times*, 97 (18): 36–37.

Wills, T. & Ford, P. (2001) Assessing older people – contemporary issues for nursing. *Nursing Older People*, 12 (9): 16–20.

Woods, R.T. (1999) Mental health problems in late life. In: R.T. Woods (ed.) *Psychological Problems of Ageing*. Chichester: John Wiley & Sons.

Chapter 13
Challenges to the Delivery
of Holistic Care

Chapter aims

> ### This chapter will:
>
> - outline some of the constraining influences on holistic practice
> - explore the organisational, educational and institutional factors influencing contemporary nursing
> - describe the interpersonal challenges nurses might encounter in attempting to meet the mental health needs of the patient
> - explore how structural support mechanisms can assist nurses in these aspects of their work.

Introduction

This book has covered a wide range of common mental health problems that might be encountered in the general hospital, the broader mental health needs of the hospital population and, most importantly, the practical skills, interventions and mechanisms required for addressing these. In some respects, there is nothing particularly new or startling in any of the chapters. The authors have gathered together the best of the relevant evidence and literature and, adding their own perspective, fashioned it into a coherent whole aimed at equipping nurses with the necessary knowledge and skills, experience and confidence to make use of it.

There is a wealth of literature relating to holistic care and a long-established consensus that, conceptually, it is central to nursing. However, as this chapter suggests, there are considerable organisational, educational, financial and clinical challenges to its actual delivery. Some of these challenges are almost as long established as the consensus about its value, but some are a consequence of more recent changes in nursing and the UK health care system in which it operates. While providing a very brief overview of these challenges we shall also aim to identify systemic strategies to support nurses in overcoming them as they endeavour to meet both the physical and the mental health needs of their patients.

Impact of changes in the NHS on nursing

In many, if not all, hospitals, the reality in terms of the delivery of holistic care is some distance from that detailed in textbooks, policies and clinical guidelines. Meeting the mental health needs of patients is an aspiration for almost all nurses and nursing teams but can often seem quite remote. This book might, then, appear to propose quite radical and far-reaching changes in practice. Such change would have to occur on a number of levels but, in considering how that might be realised, it is necessary to consider the challenges involved.

Obholzer and Roberts (1994) observed, 'We would all like to believe that the world is fundamentally a logical, well-managed place' but that the evidence against this being the case is overwhelming. If true of the world, how true of the National Health Service (NHS) and what is still its clinical and ideological cornerstone, the hospital? This is a problem that has particularly vexed successive UK governments, of both political parties, since the 1980s. Partly it stemmed from the breakdown of the ideological and political consensus that had stood since 1948, and partly it was fuelled by the growing difficulty in funding it (Klein, 1989; Hart, 2004). The consequence of these concerns was a succession of re-organisations to the point where, since 1997, health authorities have been transformed firstly into primary care groups and then primary care trusts. Regional health authorities have given way to strategic health authorities and workforce confederations, which have since been merged and will be disbanded. Trusts have been merged and merged again to form huge, incredibly complex organisations employing thousands of staff.

Still, New Labour has been unable to find a formula with which it is satisfied and by 2005 had increased private sector provision of health care within the NHS to 15%. There is also a strand of contemporary thinking that has suggested the NHS would benefit from the introduction of managerial 'expertise' brought in from the private sector or elsewhere. This is despite a mountain of evidence of poor management and practice in industry, business and commercial health services (Syrett & Lammiman, 1999). Moreover, some of the modern ills of the NHS are directly traceable to ideologically driven changes that have introduced increasingly commercial and business-like managerial practices into what is still a public service. The internal market, ostensibly having been abandoned, is being re-invented in the guise of foundation trusts (Hart, 2004).

One such problem is that many contemporary nurses are ill-equipped to provide the type of holistic, patient-focused care that will meet the mental health needs of the patients in the general hospital setting. Many perceived shortcomings in nursing care are often laid at the door of individual nurses or nursing teams. However, we would hope that readers will recognise that, as is often actually the case when all of the circumstances are considered, this does not fall into this category. Nurses have limited meaningful involvement in the ideological direction of the NHS, effective control of the hospital, or in key decision-making forums on policy, funding or strategy. Yet, because nursing is at the heart of providing patient care and forms such a huge component of the NHS workforce, it encompasses all that is good about Britain's health care services but has to live with its shortcomings and problems.

Holistic care and the expanding role of the nurse

As shall be argued below, there are a range of potential strategic decisions and changes that could be made by non-nurses that would impact favourably on the broader parameters of nursing practice. Of equal importance, individuals can develop a vision of how they want to see their own nursing practice and the clinical areas in which they work develop. Making small changes has an effect. Collaborating with like-minded individuals, or teams, can spread the impact of those changes and gradually create a genuine difference at an organisational level. Many nurses working in hospitals are very aware of the need to take a holistic perspective and use it as the basis of their care, some are in a position to use their knowledge and skills, while others, given the opportunity, would gladly do so. Nor is it possible to generalise too far. Even in individual hospitals, there is a tremendous variation in practice, with some ward teams and units adopting a more progressive approach to providing for the mental health needs of their patients. These exemplify the potential to establish best practice in their own individual areas, and reflect the opportunities when nurses and other clinicians take the needs of the patient as their starting point rather than organisational priorities and centralised policy directives.

However, there is a need to recognise that such clinical work is not without its own difficulties. Continuing emotional intimacy with patients who are seriously ill and perhaps dying can provoke high levels of anxiety, prompting a range of psychological and emotional defences. Without adequate support, this can become an increasingly dysfunctional process for the individual and, as the anxiety and distress is unresolved and displaced, for the institution (Menzies, 1970; Dartington, 1994). Thus the culture of being 'busy' with physical tasks and care can serve as an apparently valid alternative to spending time with patients in ways in which a greater level of emotional intimacy becomes inevitable (Harrison, 2003). Moreover, well intentioned organisational priorities such as early discharge and even the increased role of specialist practitioners all impact upon this. New approaches to care can easily be viewed as potentially more challenging; limited attention may be paid to the idea that a more proactive approach to the broader care process may in fact prove effective, both in terms of improving patient outcomes and the use of nurses' time, rather than simply being yet another demand upon the practitioner. A lack of confidence, perceived lack of skills and un-acknowledged anxieties when taking responsibility for addressing a person's mental health needs can all feed into this (Caplan, 1964).

None of this can be transformed in isolation: nurses require the safety net of coherent clinical supervision, cohesive teamwork and consistent boundaries, as well as structured mechanisms to address and resolve organisational problems and the issues they find stressful. Other factors that can be introduced to facilitate a more holistic approach are outlined in Box 13.1.

Box 13.1 Summary of the factors that can facilitate nurses in addressing the psychosocial needs of the patient.

Integrating different elements of nursing care, including those carried out by specialist staff, e.g. diabetes specialists, discharge co-ordinators, etc. This can be achieved by having ward nurses working alongside them while they carry out specialist assessments and/or procedures and ensuring key nursing staff are fully aware of what has been happening via a verbal and written report

Using relationship building skills (see Chapter 1) more acutely from the outset, recognising the challenge posed by shorter hospital stays for patients. One simple way in which this can be done is by making a primary nursing system work effectively or, at least, maintaining the 'named nurse' system of allocating the same nurse to patients on a consistent basis (Ersser & Tutton, 1991)

Increasing awareness of how to make use of nursing models that acknowledge the psychological needs of the patient in practice and facilitate psychosocial interventions

As a nursing and multi-professional team, acknowledging the importance of the patient's psychological, social and emotional needs, and identifying how individual nurses can incorporate meeting these into their programme of care for the patient. This may mean identifying tasks that nurses will no longer be involved in (which are usually non-nursing in nature anyway), and ways in which these can be undertaken by other staff

For ward nurses to recognise the relationship between physical and psychological factors, and between a patient's psychological state and behaviour. This can emphasise the value in helping patients with their psychological, social and emotional needs, and that they actually have the necessary skills to do this

For the organisational and administrative burdens to be rationalised, allowing nurses more time in the clinical area, i.e. the importance of clinical work being given greater recognition organisationally.

Difficulties encountered by contemporary nurses in the provision of holistic care

One of the reasons there is such a wide variation in how nurses and clinical teams address mental health care is the historical separation of mind and body (Turp, 2001), which led to the development of physically orientated health services, and those that were focused on mental and psychiatric care. Despite laudable aims and a certain degree of rhetoric, there is still little evidence of successful commissioning, planning and integration of mental health and physical (acute) care services (Department of Health (DoH), 2001c; Sherratt & Younger-Ross, 2004). It is arguable that nurses practising holistic care would be in a position to draw these together more coherently. However, their relative lack of strategic influence and exclusion from forums which shape services or their professional needs, means that these remain subordinated to those of the medical profession, the wider organisational needs of their own institutions and the NHS.

Giving nurses a greater role in decision-making and developing a philosophy of care, at once both more holistic and more integrated, would clearly have benefits for the patient and for nursing and nurses. However, it is less an option than a necessity. Hospitals, once derided by some critics as 'health factories' (Carpenter, 1988) are rapidly becoming illness factories, paying little attention to the positive aspects of the health of patients, or even continuity of care. Nurses can only have a very limited future in this brave new world. If nursing is reduced to a series of technical or – worse – mechanistic tasks, there is a very real risk that future governments facing escalating economic pressures and 'difficult choices' will take the view that anyone can carry these out, especially if they are willing to do it for less money.

Yet the current government, like every other before it, stresses its commitment to the NHS in general and nurses particularly, decorating its 'You never had it so good,' message with a dazzling array of not very illuminating statistics. Nurses are rarely convinced, however, and though the current New Labour government can rightly boast of having increased the funding of the NHS by more than 25%, many analysts have demonstrated how this is insufficient both for the demands being made of the service and to match the government's own ambitions for it (Kellner, 1999). New Labour's claim that it has increased the number of nurses working in the NHS during its period of office is supported by the evidence, as collated by the Department of Health (www.dh.gov.uk), which shows there has been an increase in the number of both individual nurses and whole time equivalents since 1997.[1]

---

[1] Individual nurses may actually be working part time. Computing the numbers in whole time equivalents effectively adds together all such posts, as well as those where the post holder is working a full week, and illustrates the equivalent of how many full time staff are employed, a far more reliable and consistent measure than actual people in post.

This, however, only serves to highlight the paradox of the recent policy agenda, as many nurses feel more hard pressed than ever whereas expenditure on temporary staff in the NHS soared to £810 million in 2000–01 with one in ten trusts spending over 20% of its wage bill on temporary staff (Mulholland, 2001). These apparent contradictions are not irreconcilable. Many of the additional nursing posts are swallowed up by nurses moving into new areas of work such as walk-in centres, home treatment teams or NHS Direct. Moreover, many of the nurses drawn to such services are often very experienced and leave a 'quality gap' in the services from which they depart, and the overall value and cost effectiveness of such 'modernisation' remains unproved (Hart, 2004).

In fact, nursing has changed so much since the mid-nineteenth century that it is difficult to compare different epochs. Contemporary nurses can, nonetheless, rightly claim to be facing new and wide ranging challenges to their role and status. In the past two decades, in addition to the major re-organisations already quoted above, there has been a new grading system for nurses, which was then abandoned for *Agenda for Change*; nursing's ruling body has been overhauled and renamed; a new system for the education and training of nurses introduced; and, since New Labour came to office, a policy revolution. Nurses have not gained any significant influence on the policy agenda, either locally within their own hospitals, or nationally (Hart, 1994). In this context, the provision of holistic care has been a casualty.

All of these changes will, however, have a major impact on nursing and nurses with most, if not all, being wrapped up in the language of 'modernisation'. Critics of health and nursing policy thus risk the accusation of defending old and outmoded practices, while ideologically motivated 'modernisers' claim they are only seeking 'progress'. Yet the process has failed to engage nurses as an occupational group, to the extent that few are aware of, or have any interest in, the detail of policies such as *The NHS Plan* (DoH, 2000), *Making a Difference* (DoH, 1999) or even *Improving Working Lives* (DoH, 2001a). In part, this is because they have little sense of ownership with such policies. But it also reveals how little direct impact the policies actually make on their work and patient care. In language and tone they often seem divorced from the day-to-day reality experienced by nurses on the wards. This is not to suggest that policy is unimportant or that nurses should ignore either that or the political decisions that shape them. Indeed, it should be recognised that these are the decision-making constructs that mediate the environment and structures within which nurses work. Moreover, any lack of confidence in those structures or sense of grievance about the nature of the work will, at some stage, require more than local initiatives to address them (Hart, 2004).

The expanded role of the nurse has been portrayed as a cornerstone of the 'modernised' NHS (DoH, 1999). Its merits and drawbacks have been much debated (see, for example, Salvage & Smith, 2000). However, few commentators appear to have recognised that it is as much a myth as was its nineteenth century equivalent, the 'suitable woman' who symbolised the change from the untrained, unregulated 'Sarah Gamps' to the new Nightingale nurses. Nor is there anything new or 'modern' to the expansion of the parameters of nursing. It was very much a feature of late nineteenth century nursing as nurses began to take on some of the duties jealously guarded by the physician until technology, medical advances and their dominance of the health market necessitated changes in the doctor's own role (Gamarnikov, 1991). This continued throughout the twentieth century, perhaps reaching its apotheosis as the nursing process that had replaced task allocation metamorphosed into primary nursing (Ersser & Tutton, 1991). However, nineteenth century nurses were abandoning domestic tasks to take on new nursing duties; the contemporary nurse is often relinquishing elements that were once considered integral to the nursing role in order to take on different areas of work that identify their newer role as 'special' or specialist.

As was the case for earlier generations of nurses, the current changes are intrinsically linked to the division of labour between nurses and doctors and reflect the subordination of the nursing role to that of their medical colleagues.[2] Key drivers in changing current nursing practice have been new policy initiatives such as national service frameworks, the introduction of personal medical services and new contracts for general practitioners (GPs) and consultants, reductions in the hours junior doctors can work, as well as a host of changes in medical and surgical practice.

In this respect, while the parameters of nursing might be expanding, the actual role of many nurses is narrowing. In order to take on new tasks it is inevitable that specialist nurses like discharge co-ordinators, outreach critical care nurses and diabetes specialists have had to abandon the emphasis on 'the holism of patient health promotion, maintenance and restoration' (Royle & Walsh, 1992) and nurturing any continuing relationship with the patient that would underpin it. They can also take away from ward nurses many aspects of the work that would have been routine only a few years ago. Nor is the taking on of reductionist tasks likely to provide the increased status politicians and managers claim it will give to nursing and the 'professionalist' wing of nursing hopes will finally be achieved (Hart, 2004). Moreover, at the same time the Department of Health identifies a lack of attention to nursing care and responsibilities as being distressing to patients and a source

---

[2] There are, however, complex layers to this widely accepted position. Although there is a wealth of evidence, already referenced here, which supports the notion of a subordinated nursing workforce, a closer examination of literature – both primary and secondary – throughout the past 150 years amply demonstrates one of nursing's greatest strengths, which is the ability of nursing to subvert forms of authority and develop its agenda using persuasion, non-confrontational methods or artful manipulation of the 'system' and those in power (Hart, 2004). Perhaps this offers one of the greatest hopes that nurses working in areas where there are no organisational initiatives or policies for meeting the mental health needs of patients can develop systems, relationships and initiatives of their own.

of serious concern. Additionally, government targets can reflect the flawed strategy of prescribing care through a heavily centralised policy agenda if they impinge on the nurse–patient relationship. The demand for all patients to be discharged from the emergency department within fours hours of arrival is, on the face of it, highly desirable. When it becomes apparent, however, that the reality of this is that it can leave nurses having neither the time nor the opportunity to provide all aspects of the patient's care because of managerial pressure to move the patient out of the department, it becomes less clear whether or not the correct target has been set, or if nursing is valued as an intrinsic intervention in itself. Similarly, nurses in walk-in centres were expected to provide holistic assessments and care for patients that would be qualitatively different from the time-limited consultations patients experienced with GPs. Yet these, too, were sacrificed as targets were increased for the numbers of patients to be seen in a day.

Achieving holistic care for the patient in the modern NHS

Holistic care, if it is practised, has an enormous impact upon the hospital. Cultivating a meaningful relationship with patients and attending to their health needs takes time and can result in conflicts with other organisational needs and demands. For example, with a limited number of beds and huge demand, there is a simple equation related to admissions and discharges. Genuinely seeking to meet all of the patient's health needs, however, might result in patients having longer hospital stays, completely different nursing care and would transform the position of nursing in the hospital hierarchy. To do so would not only test the organisation but also challenge the skills, knowledge and experience of nurses uneducated in, and unaccustomed to, such an approach.

It is hard to imagine any hospital or clinical team ever reaching a position where it would renounce the principles of holistic care. Not only would it be politically difficult but many would argue that it would not make clinical sense or fit with the wider ethos and objectives of health care provision in the twenty-first century. This means the work to begin to resolve the tensions and challenges outlined in this chapter becomes even more pressing. A range of potential solutions has been outlined throughout this book, aimed at changing practice at the individual, institutional and even national level. Perhaps the overriding view of the authors here is that individual nurses must be included in the process and empowered, within given parameters, to make the changes they see as applicable and necessary. Although this is a view that the government has enshrined in policies such as *Improving Working Lives* (DoH, 2001a) and *Shifting the Balance of Power* (DoH, 2001b), these have yet to make an impact at the level of decision-making, and nurses' involvement in shaping strategy and service configuration. However, the mechanisms are available, as are structural approaches such as shared governance (DoH, 2001b).

There is no single formula for shared governance because its agenda must be generated by the workforce. Nonetheless, elements of its composition in the NHS relevant to the implementation of holistic care would need to include:

- identifying appropriate means for communications for different areas and staff groups
- identifying key areas for information giving, consultation, negotiation and devolved decision-making – and staying with the process and results
- identifying local rewards and performance incentives for the implementation of change and meeting desired patient outcomes
- minimising the policy agenda to key performance areas, with a degree of local autonomy monitored from the centre, for meeting simplified, broader and more realistic clinical targets
- developing new decision-making models, both clinical and organisational, using a problem-solving approach
- developing openness, critical thinking and well managed risk-taking
- initiating a programme of clinical supervision for all nurses
- looking at the use of time for nurses and other staff, with the aim of increasing but managing the amount of time nurses spend with patients
- utilising a formula of nurse–patient allocation such as primary nursing, aimed at quantifying the staff resource available for patients and using the nurse–patient relationship as the focus of care
- developing leadership and role modelling through mentorship and supervision
- personal development planning
- continuing education and training programmes focusing on the skills outlined in Chapter 1.

In taking a holistic approach to the organisation and delivery of treatment and care, we take a major step forward in making holistic care for individual patients, incorporating their mental health needs with the physical, a consistent and widespread reality.

References

Caplan, G. (1964) *Principles of Preventative Psychiatry*. New York: Basic Books.

Carpenter, M. (1988) *Working for Health*. London: Routledge.

Dartington, A. (1994) Where angels fear to tread: idealism, despondency and inhibition in thought in hospital nursing. In: A. Obholzer & V.Z. Roberts (eds) *The Unconscious at Work: individual and organisational stress in the human services*. London: Routledge.

Department of Health (1999) *Making a Difference*. London: DoH.

Department of Health (2000) *The NHS Plan*. London: DoH.

Department of Health (2001a) *Improving Working Lives*. London: DoH.

Department of Health (2001b) *Shifting the Balance of Power*. London: DoH.

Department of Health (2001c) *Caring for Older People. A Nursing Priority: report of the standing Nursing and Midwifery Advisory Committee*. London: DoH.

Ersser, S. & Tutton, E. (eds) (1991) *Primary Nursing in Perspective*. Middlesex: Scutari Press.

Gamarnikov, E. (1991) Nurse or woman: gender and professionalism in reformed nursing 1860–1923. In: P. Holden & J. Littlewood (eds) *Anthropology and Nursing*. London: Routledge.

Harrison, A. (2003) Are we really too busy to care? *Nursing Times*, 99 (33): 17.

Hart, C. (1994) *Behind the Mask: nurses, their unions and nursing policy*. London: Baillière Tindall.

Hart, C. (2004) *Nurses and Politics: the impact of power and practice*. Basingstoke: Palgrave Macmillan.

Kellner, P. (1999) £40 billion is not enough for us to feel good. *The Standard*, 1 February.

Klein, R. (1989) *The Politics of the NHS*, 2nd edn. London: Longman.

Menzies, I.E.P. (1970) *The Functioning of Social Systems as a Defence Against Anxiety*. London: Tavistock.

Mulholland, H. (2001) 'Chaotic' staff cover costs NHS £810 m a year. *Nursing Times*, 97 (36): 4.

Obholzer, A. & Roberts, V.Z. (1994) The troublesome individual and the troubled institution. In: A. Obholzer & V.Z. Roberts (eds) *The Unconscious at Work: individual and organisational stress in the human services*. London: Routledge.

Royle, J.A. & Walsh, M. (1992) *Watson's Medical Surgical Nursing and Related Physiology*, 4th edn. London: Baillière Tindall.

Salvage, J. & Smith, R. (2000) Who wears the trousers? *Nursing Times*, 96 (15): 24.

Sherratt, C. & Younger-Ross, S. (2004) Out of sight out of mind. *Community Care*, 29 April–5 May: 40–41.

Syrett, M. & Lammiman, J. (1999) Forget IQ – it's brains that matter. *The Observer*. 7 November.

Turp, M. (2001) *Psychosomatic Health*. Basingstoke: Palgrave Macmillan.

Website

Department of Health website – www.dh.gov.uk

Index